Busting the Diabetes Myth

Dr David Cavan is an experienced diabetes physician, based at the London Diabetes Centre and at University Hospitals Dorset. He has a passion for supporting people with diabetes and, in addition to writing books, has developed a number of self-management programmes. He currently works internationally to train health professionals, and to develop programmes to help people reverse type 2 diabetes.

www.drdavidcavan.com
 @drdavidcavan

Also by Dr David Cavan

Reverse Your Diabetes: The Step-by-Step Plan
to Take Control of Type 2 Diabetes

Reverse Your Diabetes Diet: The New Eating Plan
to Take Control of Type 2 Diabetes

Take Control of Type 1 Diabetes

The Low-Carb Diabetes Cookbook

Busting the Diabetes Myth

The Natural Way to Reverse
Type 2 Diabetes and Prediabetes

DR DAVID CAVAN

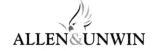

ALLEN&UNWIN

First published in trade paperback in Great Britain in 2022 by Allen & Unwin, an imprint of Atlantic Books Ltd.

Copyright © Dr David Cavan, 2022

10 9 8 7 6 5 4 3 2 1

A CIP catalogue record for this book is available from the British Library.

Trade paperback ISBN: 978 1 83895 456 7
E-book ISBN: 978 1 83895 457 4

Printed in Great Britain

Design benstudios.co.uk

Allen & Unwin
An imprint of Atlantic Books Ltd
Ormond House
26–27 Boswell Street
London
WC1N 3JZ

www.allenandunwin.com/uk

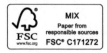

Dedicated to Mary,
my amazing wife, soulmate, counsellor
and fellow traveller

Contents

FOREWORD

A beacon of hope in a very dark world

By Dr David Unwin FRCGP, RCGP clinical expert in diabetes

I am an oldish (63 years old) GP who has looked after my local population (near Liverpool) of about 9,000 people since 1986. A few days ago I was so excited to meet my 105th patient to accomplish drug-free remission of her type 2 diabetes. That is, her blood tests showed she had non-diabetic blood sugar levels and she was no longer taking her medication for diabetes. This was a lady who only a few months ago thought her diabetes was a chronic, deteriorating condition and is now medication-free with a normal blood sugar level. She is rightly proud of her achievement! A beacon of hope in a very dark world. I agree with the author of this book, my good friend Dr David Cavan, that it is high time that the myth that type 2 diabetes is a condition that only gets worse with time was debunked.

Another pandemic.

When I started as a young GP 35 years ago there were just 57 people with diabetes in our practice; it was quite a rare illness, as was the obesity it is so often associated with. Also, it affected older people. This is important as type 2 diabetes does its damage via raised blood sugar as a function of time so older people have less time for damage to accrue. By 2012 diabetes was no longer rare – my practice had suffered an *eight-fold* increase to 472 cases! A situation made worse because the individuals were decades younger. The youngest case I have seen is just ten years old! As part of this phenomenon, amputations, heart disease and blindness had become depressingly commonplace. My answer to helping these patients was to use ever more drugs to try and reduce their blood sugar levels. Exactly the same treatment model is still occurring in practices right across the world. Yet the idea that drugs will ever be the answer to the epidemic of diabetes is another myth. In England we now spend over £600 million on drugs for diabetes each year, yet still the cases keep rising, to over four million people now having diabetes in the UK. This is a global phenomenon; another worldwide pandemic, now killing over four million people each year.

It's not just about type 2 diabetes. It may be a surprise to learn the information in this book could help with far, far more than just diabetes. For example, about 25% of adults in the developed world now have non-alcoholic fatty liver disease (NAFLD) – yet another global problem. The wonderful work of Professor Roy Taylor in 2012 showed not just how a fatty liver interfered with the work of insulin, causing so-called insulin resistance and eventually diabetes itself, but also how this and even type 2 diabetes could be reversed by a better diet and weight loss. NAFLD and type 2 diabetes are associated with yet another epidemic; central obesity (having a big belly), which is linked to the increased risk of at least eight different cancers, plus high blood pressure and cardiovascular disease.

So in addition to improving blood sugar control, if you follow Dr Cavan's advice in *Busting the Diabetes Myth* you may also see significant weight loss, better blood pressure, improved lipid profiles and liver function tests – not to mention better self-esteem! Key to achieving all this is improving your understanding of the role the hormone insulin plays in type 2 diabetes, which is explained in Chapter 2. If you have insulin resistance you will struggle to control your blood sugar – but the central and hopeful point being made here is that insulin resistance is reversible. This book explains how this can be brought about in terms the interested reader can easily understand.

I hope that by reading this well-organized, clever book you will have a far better understanding of not just the causes of type 2 diabetes but also what you may be able to do to improve diabetic control and indeed many other aspects of your health.

We have eaten our way into this epidemic of diabetes, what if we could eat our way out of it? Read this book to find out how!

Dr David Unwin FRCGP, RCGP clinical expert in diabetes

@lowcarbGP

Preface

I have worked as a diabetes specialist for over 30 years, and it is fair to say that for the first 20 of those years, managing people with type 2 diabetes was of little interest to me, unless they had developed complications that needed my specialist input. Less complex cases were managed by GPs. Until ten years ago, we believed that type 2 diabetes was an inevitably and inexorably progressive condition that would get worse as time went on, and so managing it was all rather depressing for me as a doctor. It must have been even more depressing for my patients, who were asked to make lifestyle changes and to take medication, often with unpleasant side-effects, in order to control a condition that they had been told will in any case likely progress. To make matters worse, they were advised to base all their meals on starchy carbohydrates, which meant that every time they ate, their food caused their blood sugar levels to increase, just as they were taking medication to decrease their sugar levels. It is no wonder that many who followed the advice they were given felt they were failing in some way.

All that changed about ten years ago. By then we had seen a number of new diabetes drugs come on stream, often with great hope and even more hype, but which I felt just failed to live up to expectations. I was becoming disillusioned with the use of medications to manage type 2 diabetes. At about the same time, we were beginning to learn that what we had believed about type 2 diabetes being a progressive condition was not necessarily true; that in fact it could be reversed by lifestyle change. And so, for the first time in my career, I started to ask people with type 2 diabetes about their diet and their lifestyle. I began to suggest that they ignore the official advice and strive to *reduce* the carbohydrates in their meals. Those that did found that their blood sugar levels improved and often they needed to reduce their medications. One of my early patients was visiting from Nigeria, and by changing his diet he was able to stop insulin injections, which back home were very expensive for him to buy. For the first time in my career, I became really excited about the prospect of treating people with type 2 diabetes. So much so, that when a couple of years later I was asked to write a book for people with type 2 diabetes, I leapt at the opportunity to share my new understanding and ideas, to give people hope that they could potentially reverse their condition and provide some tips as to how they could achieve it, principally by reducing the carbohydrates (sugars and starches) in their diet.

That book, *Reverse your diabetes: the step-by-step plan to take control of type 2 diabetes*, was published in 2014. To be honest, I was rather nervous about what might happen next. It was (and still is) quite rare for a diabetes specialist to write a book to advise people to ignore standard dietary advice and to consider reducing their medications. So much so that it caused quite a stir in some of the upper echelons of the diabetes establishment. Some thought I was jeopardising my reputation and my career for a fad diet. I didn't think they were right, but I didn't know for sure. I didn't have to wait long to find out. Within a few months, people contacted me to tell me that they had followed my advice and reversed their diabetes. I then began to hear about other doctors in the UK and overseas who had similar ideas and were also seeing great success with their patients. Since then, they and I have been on a journey during which our understanding about reversal or remission of type 2 diabetes has increased enormously. This journey has taken me to different countries to help doctors adopt the same approach for their patients. And you know what? My experience is that regardless of culture, race or income level, people who get the right support are able to make changes that significantly improve their health, even if they do not manage to fully reverse their condition.

Things are beginning to change. There is now greater acceptance that type 2 diabetes can be reversed, and that a low carbohydrate diet can help people achieve that. Despite this, I still come across many health professionals who are sceptical about reversal of type 2 diabetes, and so many of their patients continue to follow the old ways of managing their diabetes, oblivious that there is an alternative. They are following and believing what I now term the 'diabetes myths', and so it is my aim in this new book to show what I believe those myths to be and bust them, one by one, using the latest evidence and my own experience. As with *Reverse your diabetes*, I also include detailed explanations about how type 2 diabetes develops, the consequences of having type 2 diabetes (brought sharply into focus during the Covid-19 pandemic), and the treatments available, as I believe it is important that people with type 2 diabetes have a good understanding of their condition, so that they are fully informed when making choices as to how they want to manage it, and whether they want to try and reverse it. I have also included real life stories from people who read *Reverse your diabetes* and did just that, and from others who used different resources to reverse their diabetes.

The biggest myth is that type 2 diabetes is a progressive condition. It does not have to be, and in this book I explain what you can do to minimize the chance that it progresses and maximize the chance that it reverses. You do not have to have type 2 diabetes to benefit from this book. Prediabetes is the precursor to type 2 diabetes and if you have prediabetes, many of the same principles I put forward here will help ensure not only that you do not progress to type 2 diabetes, but also that you increase the chances that you can reverse your prediabetes and again achieve normal blood sugar levels. So, whether you have prediabetes, are newly diagnosed with type 2 diabetes, or have had type 2 diabetes for many years, my hope is that this book will help you achieve long-lasting improvements in your health and wellbeing.

PART ONE

Introduction

CHAPTER 1

You CAN do it

The biggest myth about type 2 diabetes is that it is a condition that just gets worse over time, and there's nothing you can do to stop that happening. This is a view that is firmly held by many people, including some health professionals. There is a good reason for this – we used to believe it was true. However, that was a long time ago. It is nearly 20 years since we first learnt that type 2 diabetes can be prevented, and over 10 years since we learnt it can be reversed. Stories of people reversing their diabetes are now quite common in the media, and you may well know someone who has managed to do just that. And yet, too many of my medical colleagues still treat their patients as if nothing has changed, as if what they were taught 30 years ago still takes precedence over more recent scientific advances in understanding. And if one of those people is a doctor or nurse helping you manage your diabetes or prediabetes, that can be quite disconcerting. Even Diabetes UK, which purports to represent people with diabetes, states: 'Some people can manage it through healthier eating, being more active or losing weight. But eventually most people will need medication to bring their blood sugar down to their target level.'[1] It acknowledges that some people are able to put their diabetes into remission, but it goes on to say that this is not possible for everyone. While this is true – it is not possible for everyone – the way it is presented gives a subliminal message that goes something like this: well, it is possible to reverse type 2 diabetes, but it's very difficult and most people aren't up to it, and so you will probably need medication to control it.

I often compare this rather defeatist approach with that of doctors who treat cancer. Some cancers have a very high likelihood of causing death, and yet there could be treatments that provide a small chance of achieving remission. I have personal experience of this from a few years ago, when my father was diagnosed with an aggressive form of leukaemia. It was resistant to normal treatments but there was a more complex therapy that offered the possibility of success in controlling the disease. We all understood that he was very ill, and I guess deep down I knew he would not recover, but the team looking after him focused on the positive, on the slim chance that the treatment could help him pull through. During this time, a nurse kindly and gently encouraged me to stay positive by saying to me, 'There is always hope.' Those words, and that wider focus on the positive, greatly helped me through that time, even though his condition took a turn for the worse before he was able to start the treatment, and he died shortly afterwards.

Now the chances of achieving remission of type 2 diabetes are a lot higher than my dad's chances of overcoming his illness. Yet many health professionals seem to focus on the negatives – it's hard work and most people won't manage it. However, gradually and begrudgingly, the understanding that it is possible to reverse type 2 diabetes is replacing the myth that type 2 diabetes is a condition that only gets worse. Since my last book, *Reverse Your Diabetes*, was published in 2014, there have been numerous research studies showing that many people have been able to reverse their diabetes. In addition, I have been contacted by many people who had read my book and told me with great joy how they too have been able to join the ranks of those whose diabetes is in remission. You can read some of their stories later in this book.

So what do we mean by reversal and remission of type 2 diabetes? In August 2021, an international consensus statement was published by the American Diabetes Association, the European Association for the Study of Diabetes and Diabetes UK, which defines remission as achieving non-diabetic levels of glucose in the bloodstream for at least three months, while taking no diabetes medications.[2] This is usually judged by means of a blood test of glycated haemoglobin level or HbA1c. HbA1c provides an overview of diabetes control over the previous six to eight weeks – so it is a sort of average blood glucose level. A level of 48 mmol/mol (millimoles per mole – the standard way of measuring HbA1c – also represented as 6.5 per cent) or less, without using diabetes medication, indicates remission of type 2 diabetes. Remission of prediabetes is achieved if the HbA1c is maintained below 42 mmol/mol (6.0 per cent). Chapter 2 explains all this in more detail.

This statement also recommended that remission be the preferred term to reversal of diabetes. However, I like the term reversal and I also think there is a slight difference. I explain reversal as the process by which people can reverse what I call 'the diabetes disease process', which will also be explained in more detail in Chapter 2. By making lifestyle changes, people can reverse the disease process that caused their diabetes (or prediabetes). In some, the reversal will be complete, their metabolism will have normalized and they will have achieved remission; but others may reverse the process to some extent. They may lose weight, successfully reduce their doses or number of medications and achieve better control of their diabetes, but still have the condition. In other words, they could be described as having partially reversed their diabetes. They did not achieve remission, but nevertheless, they have significantly improved the outlook for their health for many years to come.

What does that mean for you? If you have recently been diagnosed with prediabetes or type 2 diabetes, there is a high likelihood that if you are able to make lifestyle changes, then you can reverse the metabolic abnormalities that drive the diabetes disease process. You might be able to reverse the condition completely, so that your diabetes is in remission, or you might be able to achieve much better control of your condition, perhaps with less need for medication. Although you will still be classed as having diabetes (or prediabetes), you will have busted the myth that type 2 diabetes is likely to get worse and require ever more medication.

If you have had type 2 diabetes or prediabetes for many years, the research suggests that complete reversal is less likely than in people who have been diagnosed more recently. However, I have known people achieve remission after many years of having type 2 diabetes, in some cases having been on insulin injections, and so can confirm that it is never too late to make lifestyle changes that will maximize the chance of reversing the disease process. Therefore, regardless of how long you have had type 2 diabetes or prediabetes, it is definitely worth considering making some changes to your lifestyle – they just might work! And with the knowledge gained during the Covid pandemic about the increased risks associated with having diabetes, it has arguably never been so important to try.

Now the fact that you are reading this book is a good start, and hopefully indicates that you are open to making some changes to improve your health. As you read on, you will gain valuable information that you can use to make choices about your diet and lifestyle to help improve your health. I deliberately used the word 'choices' there, to emphasize that any process of lifestyle change is by definition your choice, and yours alone. In this book I will provide advice – not insist you make sudden and radical changes to what you eat or how you live. My goal is to provide you with information that will offer you good options, and then it is up to you to decide whether you want to make any changes, which changes you want to make and when you want to make them. The whole point of lifestyle change is to make changes that will be long-lasting. They therefore have to be changes that are sustainable in the long term. That means you have to be fully on board with – and committed to making – those changes.

And the changes you make are not for my benefit or your doctor's benefit or anyone else's benefit. They are solely for your benefit. So rather than just coming up with a list of changes that you think you should make, or that you feel you would like to make, I suggest that, first of all, you consider why you want to make changes – in other words, what it is that you want to achieve in respect of your health. That is what I call goal-setting.

You see, just like those colleagues of mine who tend to focus on the negative, you too may be experiencing similar negative feelings. Maybe you have had diabetes for many years, and have tried to 'follow the rules' but always found that your glucose levels are too high. Maybe you have just been diagnosed with diabetes, but have struggled with being overweight for much longer. Perhaps you have tried different diets, maybe managed to shed a few pounds, but it was hard work, and you ended up back at square one. Maybe you have come to accept you will always be overweight, or unhealthy, as if you have constructed your own myths. That would be quite understandable. It would also be understandable if you felt cynical about your ability to turn things around, to bust your own myths.

However, I am inviting you to focus on something else – not on the negatives, however much they have been part of your experience. Rather, focus on the positives – the 'what ifs'. Growing numbers of people in many countries have experienced the positive life-changing effect of reversing their diabetes or prediabetes. They have proved to themselves that it is possible and they are enjoying life in a way that just a short while ago they could not have imagined. Reversing diabetes is possible. Losing a lot of weight is possible. Regaining the energy you had 20 years ago is possible. Being able to reduce or stop medications for diabetes is possible. Doing away with tablets for high blood pressure, pain, erectile dysfunction, gout and heartburn is possible. I have had patients who have been able to come off medications for all of these conditions. Now, I never make promises to people about what will be achievable for them, as this depends hugely on how their body responds to the changes they are able to make, but I can say that, if you are able to follow the advice in this book, there is a high likelihood of improving your health and wellbeing in some – or many – of these ways.

I have already mentioned that the changes that will help restore your health need to be long term. Not a short, sharp shock, not a crash diet, but forever. Changing what, when or how you eat, will by definition mean changing long-held habits, many of which will be so ingrained into your daily life that you may not realize quite why you eat what you do, when you do. It is possible – indeed very likely – that, after following a new way of eating for several months, at some point you will find yourself back with your old habits, either because you slip into autopilot without realizing or because you have hit a difficult time. Life has a habit of throwing a spanner in the works, often with no warning and often when you least expect it. When that happens, you will need to get yourself back on track and remotivate yourself, so it helps to have in mind some really good reasons for getting back on track.

Which brings me back to your goal. When setting your goal, allow yourself to think, dream even, about what you would like to achieve in respect of improving your health – not only 'what' but also 'why'. For example, if your goal is to lose a lot of weight, rather than thinking about that as just reversing a negative ('I will no longer be overweight'), focus on some positives that will happen if you do lose weight, such as being able to climb stairs without getting out of breath, being able to play around with the kids, getting into clothes you haven't been able to wear for years or taking up a sport you used to enjoy. If your goal is to reverse your diabetes, how would that make you feel? Apart from not having to take medications, picture regaining the energy you no longer have and being able to think more clearly. Essentially, imagine the new you.

So, before going any further, I encourage you to ask yourself the questions overleaf, and to write the answers down, either in this book or in a separate notebook. Take some time to really think about them, as we will refer back to your answers as you progress through the book. Maybe you do not feel you can answer all the questions just yet. That's fine. You can also change your answers at any time. We will return to the questions again in Chapter 11. But before reading any further, have a go now:

1. What frustrates you most about your health at present?

2. How do you want things to be different?

3. How will you feel when you have achieved this?

4. What is your main goal – the thing you would like to achieve from reading this book?

Identifying your main goal will help you focus not only on the benefits you can look forward to as you achieve it, but also on the changes that you need to make in order to achieve it. In Chapter 11, we will explore how you can set yourself smaller goals representing the changes that will help you work towards your main goal.

Depending on how quickly you read, it may be a little while before you finish this book. So, right at the start, I want to set out some steps that you can take immediately that will help reduce your glucose levels, get you feeling better and set you on the path to reversing the diabetes disease process. I call this my diabetes 'first aid' guide – simple steps that anyone can take. You may not feel that they all apply to you, but I would encourage you to look at the list opposite and choose one or two changes that fit with your own goal and that you feel you could make immediately:

First aid guide to taking control of type 2 diabetes

Drinks

1. Stop using sugar in tea or coffee (use sweeteners if necessary).
2. Avoid sweet drinks, such as fruit juice, smoothies, squashes and fizzy drinks (drink water or sugar-free drinks as far as possible).
3. Cut down the amount of alcohol you consume, especially drinks containing carbohydrate, such as beer, cider or sweet wines.

Food

1. Avoid sweet foods, such as cakes, biscuits, jam, sweets or chocolate.
2. Eat less potatoes, rice, pasta and bread.
3. Eat more fresh green and salad vegetables.
4. Limit fresh fruit to one or two small pieces a day.

Physical activity

1. If you can, go for a 15-minute walk every day.
2. Use stairs instead of lifts or escalators.
3. Walk or cycle instead of using the car or bus for short journeys.
4. If you use a bus, get off one or two stops before your destination.

These tips reflect the key elements of managing type 2 diabetes in the short term: eating less sugar and starchy food and becoming more active. We will cover these in more detail later in the book but making one or two of these changes now will make a big difference to most people newly diagnosed with type 2 diabetes.

So, please do try to make some changes, however small. If you do not feel you can make any changes right now, you may wish to set yourself a target of one change you feel you could realistically make in the next two weeks. Please do not wait until you 'know it all' before making a start. Any changes you make now can be fine-tuned at any time as you go along.

As you make changes, you will hopefully begin to see some improvements quite quickly – in your blood glucose levels and your feeling of wellbeing. Taking control of your diabetes in this way will be the first step towards reversing your diabetes. We will discuss this in more detail later in the book (Chapter 5), but for now the message is that anything you can do to reduce your weight and your blood glucose levels will start the process of reversing the changes in your body that led to type 2 diabetes or prediabetes. And this will lead to a healthier future.

CHAPTER 2

What are prediabetes and type 2 diabetes?

A history of diabetes

The technical name of the condition is diabetes mellitus, which when translated from the Latin literally means 'passing honey' – so-called because the urine contains glucose and tastes sweet. It is thought that the condition was first described – three and a half thousand years ago in ancient Egypt – as a disease where urine was too plentiful. Then in 1,000 BC, the ancient Indian physician Sushruta described the urine being sweet, and wrote that ants and flies were attracted to it, but he thought that diabetes was a disease of the urinary tract (kidneys and bladder). He wrote that it could be inherited or develop as a result of dietary excess or obesity (perhaps referring to type 1 and type 2 diabetes). The recommended treatment was exercise. It would take until the 17th century before it was discovered that the urine was sweet because it contained sugar and that diabetes was a disease of the pancreas rather than the kidneys. In 1797, the Scottish military surgeon John Rollo heated the urine of patients until a sugary cake was all that remained. He noted that the volume of the cake increased if the patient ate bread, grains and fruit (high in carbohydrate), but decreased if he or she ate meat and poultry (low in carbohydrate). Demonstrating that there is rarely anything new in the universe, he went on to describe the case of a Captain Meredith who took to a diet low in carbohydrate and high in fat and protein. His weight fell from 224 pounds (102 kg) to 162 pounds (73 kg) and his health improved. At the time, diabetes was reported as being relatively rare and associated with wealth.

At the end of the 19th century, the role of insulin became understood. In 1889, two German physicians working jointly at the University of Strasbourg – Joseph von Mering and Oskar Minkowski – removed the pancreas from dogs. They noticed that this caused the unfortunate animals to urinate frequently on the floor – despite being previously house trained. Testing the urine, they found high levels of sugar, thus establishing a link between the pancreas and diabetes. This was then reversed by the transplantation of small pieces of the pancreas back into the dog's abdomen.

Piece by piece, the puzzle was being assembled, and by the 1920s it was established that diabetes is characterized by an excess of sugar (glucose) in the blood, resulting in glucose in the urine. The disease was often seen in overweight people in whom it could be controlled by adopting a low-carbohydrate diet. In others, insulin, extracted from animal pancreases and given by injection, led to a fall in blood glucose levels.

Types of diabetes

By the 1970s, it had become clear that there were two distinct types of diabetes:

1. **Type 1 diabetes** usually occurs first in children or young adults. It comes on quite suddenly with marked symptoms, such as thirst and weight loss, and can only be treated by insulin injections.

2. **Type 2 diabetes** usually occurs in later life and it has become increasingly clear that it is related to our modern lifestyles, characterized by unhealthy food and physical inactivity. Its onset is usually far more gradual, without any specific symptoms, and it is sometimes first diagnosed by a blood test done as part of a general check-up.

There are also rare types of diabetes that occur in young people (known as maturity-onset diabetes of the young or MODY). These are inherited conditions that are not associated with weight gain, and there is usually a strong family history of diabetes. Although they mainly present in childhood, most cases can be controlled with tablets rather than insulin like type 1 diabetes.

It has also become apparent that the distinction between type 1 and type 2 diabetes is not as clear-cut as previously thought, and for people who are diagnosed in their forties and fifties, there may be a period of uncertainty before one can definitively distinguish between the two. For example, some overweight adults with type 2 diabetes present quite suddenly with very high glucose levels and require insulin at diagnosis, just like someone with type 1 diabetes. Unlike a person with type 1 diabetes, however, insulin can often be stopped once their condition stabilizes. Conversely, there is a kind of type 1 diabetes that occurs in middle-aged or older people, sometimes referred to as latent autoimmune diabetes of adulthood or LADA. As with type 1 diabetes, people with this condition are not overweight, but the onset is more like type 2 diabetes and they may be treated with tablets (see Chapter 13) for a period. However, within a few years, it becomes clear that tablets are not sufficient to control their blood glucose levels and they need insulin. From that time, their treatment is the same as for someone with type 1 diabetes. This 'overlap' between type 1 and type 2 diabetes can result in some people being given the wrong diagnosis and possibly therefore the wrong treatment – sometimes for many years.

Gestational diabetes is a condition in which diabetes occurs during pregnancy. It is similar to type 2 diabetes and is usually managed with dietary change, at least initially, although some people do need medication. It generally reverses once the baby is born, but both the mother and the baby are at increased risk of developing type 2 diabetes in later life.

Diabetes can also arise as a result of other diseases affecting hormones (for example, acromegaly, which is a condition caused by the presence of too much growth hormone, or Cushing's disease, which is caused by the presence of too much steroid hormone, cortisol). These cases are called secondary diabetes and generally reverse once the underlying condition has been treated. Cortisol is the body's natural steroid, which is released into the bloodstream at times of stress. It increases blood glucose levels to provide additional energy. Constantly high levels of cortisol can mean the body is unable to produce enough insulin to counter the effect on blood glucose levels, leading to diabetes. People who have been treated with steroids for long periods of time for conditions such as asthma may also develop diabetes. Diabetes also occurs if other diseases affect the pancreas or if the pancreas has been wholly or partly removed by surgery.

While some parts of this book may be helpful to people with other types of diabetes, it is intended specifically for people with prediabetes and type 2 diabetes, to help them learn how to manage – and potentially reverse – their condition. My book *Take Control of Type 1 Diabetes* provides advice for people with that condition.

Making a diagnosis of diabetes

The typical symptoms of diabetes include excessive urination, excessive thirst, tiredness, blurred vision, weight loss and infections such as thrush. These usually only arise once the glucose in the blood has reached a high level and the kidneys try to excrete the excess glucose in the urine. This explains why glucose can be detected in the urine and its sugary nature provides an ideal environment for the growth of bacteria and fungi, which leads to urinary infections and thrush (candidiasis). In order to excrete glucose, the kidneys need to excrete a larger volume of water (otherwise you would be peeing out sugar lumps) and this leads to dehydration, which in turn leads to excessive thirst. High glucose levels in the eyes leads to blurred vision.

In many cases of type 2 diabetes, people are diagnosed with no or only very mild symptoms. This is because diabetes is being picked up very early as a result of screening blood tests in people who do not yet have any symptoms of the disease. In other cases, people may have had diabetes for some time, which has not been diagnosed. In these cases, blood glucose levels may rise high enough for some of these symptoms to occur.

Diabetes is diagnosed by blood tests. This means that if you have symptoms which you think may be due to diabetes but the blood tests are normal, you do not have diabetes. On the other hand, if your blood tests are diagnostic of diabetes, then you have diabetes, even if you do not have any symptoms.

Diabetes can be diagnosed by a measurement of random blood glucose or fasting blood glucose, by a glucose tolerance test or by an HbA1c test. This can make it very confusing to understand what 'your numbers' mean. Furthermore, different units are used in different countries, and for prediabetes, there are also different definitions in different countries. Confused? I often am. That's why I will explain each test in some detail.

Random blood glucose test
This is often the first test that will be done and can be performed at any time of the day after breakfast. In the UK and many countries, the result is expressed as the amount of glucose molecules per litre of blood – usually expressed in terms of millimoles per litre (mmol/l). In the US and some other countries, the units are milligrams per decilitre (mg/dl). They are interpreted as shown in Table 1.

Table 1: Interpretations of random blood glucose test results

Random blood glucose*	Normal	Prediabetes	Diabetes
mmol/l	Less than 7.8	7.8–11.1	Above 11.1
mg/dl	Less than 140	140–200	Above 200

* Also applicable for the two-hour glucose tolerance test (see below).

If the random blood glucose level is normal, it is unlikely that the person has diabetes; however, if it is in the prediabetes range, then a fasting glucose or HbA1c test can be performed.

Fasting blood glucose test
This is a blood test taken after a fast of 12 hours, during which time only water can be taken by mouth. The test is generally performed

first thing in the morning. The results are interpreted as shown in Table 2.

Table 2: Interpretations of fasting blood glucose test results

Fasting blood glucose	Normal	Prediabetes*	Diabetes
mmol/l	Less than 5.5	5.5–7.0	Above 7.0
mg/dl	Less than 100	100–125	Above 125

* Note that the World Health Organization (WHO) does not recognize the term 'prediabetes' as a clinical state. Rather, it defines two separate conditions that are broadly equivalent to prediabetes. These are impaired glucose tolerance and impaired fasting hyperglycaemia, as shown in Table 2. However, if that isn't complicated enough, the WHO defines impaired fasting hyperglycaemia as a glucose level of between 6.1 and 7 mmol/l (110–125 mg/dl), whereas prediabetes is often defined as a fasting blood glucose of between 5.5 and 7.0 mmol/l (100-125 mg/dl).

If both the fasting and random blood glucose levels are normal, then the person does not have diabetes.

Glucose tolerance test

This used to be regarded as the gold standard method for diagnosing diabetes. It has now largely been superseded by HbA1c measurement but for the sake of completeness I have included it as it is still sometimes used. The glucose tolerance test (GTT) is a standardized test where a fasting blood glucose level is measured and then the person is asked to drink a liquid that contains 75 g of glucose. A further blood test is taken two hours after the drink to see how high the glucose level has risen. The results are interpreted in the same way as the fasting and random tests above. If either the fasting OR the two-hour values are diagnostic, then the person has diabetes. In other words, both have to be normal to exclude the diagnosis.

Glycated haemoglobin (HbA1c) test

When the level of blood glucose is higher than normal, the excess glucose attaches to a number of different molecules in the body. For example, when glucose attaches to the lens of the eye, it can lead to the development of cataracts, or if it attaches to soft tissue in the shoulder it may lead to a frozen shoulder. This process of attachment is termed glycation. Red blood cells contain haemoglobin, which is the substance that carries oxygen in the blood cells to the different tissues around the body and gives blood its red colour. A small amount of haemoglobin in each blood cell is glycated and just how much will depend on the amount of glucose present in the bloodstream. Red blood cells last for about four months before they are 'recycled', and the amount of glycated haemoglobin in any one cell gradually increases over this time, according to the level of glucose in the blood. Blood glucose levels change constantly according to food intake and activity levels, and so a single measurement is of little use in monitoring diabetic control. The level of glycated haemoglobin (abbreviated as HbA1c), on the other hand, is used to assess glucose levels over a longer period of time, and for many years has been the gold standard means of assessing diabetic control.

Since 2011, HbA1c has become a recognized means of diagnosing type 2 diabetes. Its measurement involves a simple blood test that can be taken at any time of day (as it reflects glucose control over the past six to eight weeks). Historically, HbA1c was expressed as the percentage of haemoglobin that was glycated. In 2011, a new system of units was introduced, which expresses the glycated component as a concentration of the total haemoglobin (millimoles per mole or mmol/mol). However, old habits die hard, and some people still refer to the old percentages. Furthermore, in some countries, the newer units haven't caught on at all. I will therefore present both units in this book. In people without diabetes, HbA1c is generally below 42 mmol/mol (6.0 per cent). An International Expert Committee has defined a result between 42 and 48 mmol/mol (6.0 and 6.5 per cent) as indicative of prediabetes,[3] and the UK and many other countries follow this definition. However, in the US and other countries that follow their guidance, prediabetes is defined as an HbA1c between 40 and 48 mmol/mol (5.7 and 6.5 per cent). Thankfully, all are agreed that a measurement of 48 mmol/mol (6.5 per cent) or above is diagnostic of type 2 diabetes. That said, it is important to be aware that a level below this does not rule out diabetes, and if there is any doubt then a glucose tolerance test should be performed. The HbA1c tests are summarized in Table 3.

Table 3: Interpretations of HbA1c test results

HbA1c (international expert definition)	Normal	Prediabetes	Diabetes
mmol/mol	Less than 42	42–48	Above 48
%	Less than 6.0	6.0–6.5	Above 6.5
HbA1c (international expert definition)			
mmol/mol	Less than 40	40–48	Above 48
%	Less than 5.7	5.7–6.5	Above 6.5

Glycated haemoglobin is also the test used to monitor control of diabetes, to ensure that the recommended treatment (lifestyle changes and medication) is achieving the desired effect. Generally, a level of 50 mmol/mol (6.7 per cent) or below is indicative of good control of diabetes; levels much above 65 mmol/mol (8 per cent) significantly increase the risk of developing diabetes-related complications.

If you have prediabetes and are able to reduce your HbA1c to below 42 mmol/mol or 6.0 per cent (40 mmol/mol or 5.7 per cent in the US!) and keep it there for at least three months, the prediabetes is said to be in remission. Similarly, if you have type 2 diabetes and maintain your HbA1c below 48 mmol/mol (6.5 per cent) for at least three months, without any medication, then your diabetes is said to be in remission.

The role of insulin in keeping glucose levels under control

In order to understand why glucose levels rise in people with prediabetes or diabetes, it is important to understand how insulin controls glucose when everything is working normally.

Glucose is a type of sugar that is used for energy by nearly all types of cells in the body and it is essential that all parts of the body have a steady supply of glucose. This glucose is obtained from the food we eat: all carbohydrates (sugars and starches) that we eat are broken down into glucose, which is then absorbed from the gut into the bloodstream so that it can be carried to the tissues and used as energy. Any spare glucose is taken up into the muscles and liver where it is stored in the form of glycogen. Glycogen in the muscles is then available for later use if the muscles need extra energy (for example, during intensive exercise). Once the glycogen stores are full, any excess glucose is converted to fat and stored in the liver.

While glucose only enters the body when we eat or drink, the body's cells require a constant supply of glucose in order to function properly. The liver, which releases some of its stored glucose into the bloodstream, provides this service and ensures that just the right amount of glucose is available during periods when we are not eating (overnight, for example). In a person without diabetes the amount of glucose in the bloodstream is kept at around 4–6 mmol/l (70–100 mg/dl).

The level of glucose in the bloodstream is controlled by insulin. Insulin is a hormone produced by the pancreas – an organ that sits just below the ribcage, behind the stomach. Like many of the body's organs, the pancreas does a lot of different things, but it has two main functions. One is to produce enzymes that are released directly into the small intestine in order to break down food so it can be absorbed into the bloodstream. These enzymes include: amylase, which breaks down starch into glucose; lipase, which breaks down fat; and protease, which breaks down proteins.

The other main function of the pancreas is to produce hormones. These are chemicals that are released into the bloodstream, and which have effects all around the body. Insulin is one of the hormones produced by the pancreas, and its job is to regulate the amount of glucose in the bloodstream, ensuring that cells get the right amount of glucose at all times. It does this in a number of ways:

1. When we eat a meal, the carbohydrate in the meal is converted into glucose in the gut and passes through the gut wall into the bloodstream. The body detects that the glucose level in the blood is rising and this leads to the pancreas producing additional insulin.

2. This insulin acts on individual cells to allow glucose to enter them. Insulin molecules attach to a receptor on the cell membrane that opens up to allow glucose in. Insulin is often likened to a 'key' that opens the cell's 'door' allowing glucose to enter the cell.

3. Insulin also stops the liver and muscles from releasing stored glucose into the blood; this allows spare glucose to be added to the glycogen stores.

When we are not eating, the pancreas continually produces a small amount of insulin that controls the release of glucose from the liver. In the liver, insulin acts like a tap that turns off the release of glucose from the liver. If glucose levels in the blood drop too low, then less insulin will be produced, opening the tap and allowing more glucose to be released from the liver. On the other hand, if glucose levels rise, then more insulin is produced, closing the tap and slowing down the release of glucose from the liver. These processes are illustrated in Figure 1.

Figure 1: The role of insulin in controlling blood glucose levels

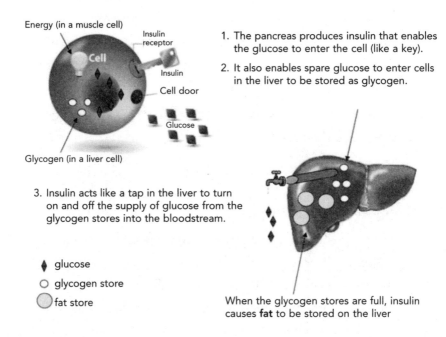

Energy (in a muscle cell)

Insulin receptor

Cell

Insulin

Cell door

Glucose

Glycogen (in a liver cell)

1. The pancreas produces insulin that enables the glucose to enter the cell (like a key).

2. It also enables spare glucose to enter cells in the liver to be stored as glycogen.

3. Insulin acts like a tap in the liver to turn on and off the supply of glucose from the glycogen stores into the bloodstream.

◆ glucose
○ glycogen store
◯ fat store

When the glycogen stores are full, insulin causes **fat** to be stored on the liver

What goes wrong in prediabetes and type 2 diabetes?

Imagine you are at a train station, waiting for a train. The train arrives and you press the button to open the doors, but the train is so packed with people that you cannot get on. If it is a busy time of day, gradually the station will become full of people unable to get onto a train.

This is a bit like what happens to glucose trying to get into the cells of a person with type 2 diabetes. In someone who has taken in more energy than they need in their food and drink, it is as if their body's cells are so full that, when insulin opens the cell doors, there is no room for the glucose to go in as it is already jam-packed.

Unlike in type 1 diabetes, where there is a complete lack of insulin (so the doors can't open), in type 2 diabetes there is insulin present, but it is ineffective in enabling glucose to enter the cells, as they are already full of glucose. So the amount of glucose in the blood increases. As the glucose levels increase, the pancreas produces more insulin to try to push the glucose into the cells. They are already full, so instead glucose is taken up into the liver where it is stored as glycogen. However, the liver can only store a certain amount of glycogen, so when the glycogen storage area is full, the excess glucose is then converted and stored in the liver as fat. Unlike glycogen, it seems that the liver can store almost unlimited amounts of fat. This would appear to be a bit of a design flaw because, when the liver becomes overrun by fat, it begins to leak glucose from the glycogen storage area. As we have read, insulin works in the liver a bit like a tap, which regulates the flow of glucose from the glycogen stores in the liver into the bloodstream in a very controlled way. However, imagine the increased pressure in those stores as a result of being squeezed by fat all around them. The tap cannot contain the pressure and the glucose leaks out and into the blood.

So, despite higher insulin levels, the glucose level in the blood increases still further. This leads to the pancreas producing more insulin, leading to more fat being stored in the liver, until eventually the body needs to find other storage areas for excess fat, including the pancreas. And just as a liver full of fat cannot work properly, a fat-filled pancreas can no longer produce insulin. And all the time the glucose in the blood increases until it passes the level for prediabetes and eventually reaches the level to diagnose type 2 diabetes. This process is shown in Figure 2.

Figure 2: How type 2 diabetes develops

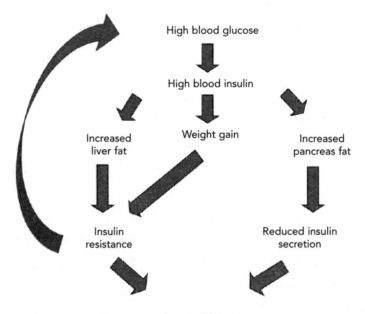

Type 2 diabetes

We saw earlier that the diagnosis of prediabetes and type 2 diabetes depends on the glucose in the blood reaching a certain level. But you can see from the above that it is clear the problem starts long before glucose levels reach the level to diagnose type 2 diabetes – or even prediabetes. This highlights how type 2 diabetes is not primarily a glucose disorder. We now understand that the main problem is with insulin, and specifically insulin resistance. This leads to high insulin levels in the bloodstream, something which can contribute to the development of high blood pressure and cholesterol levels, as well as high blood glucose levels. The implications of these changes will be discussed in Chapter 3.

Polycystic ovary syndrome (PCOS)

Another common condition associated with insulin resistance is polycystic ovary syndrome (PCOS). The WHO estimates that it affects over 3 per cent of women worldwide; other studies suggest that up to 18 per cent of women may be affected, many without having been diagnosed.

PCOS is usually diagnosed in young women and the main features are irregular or no periods, excess body or facial hair, having acne and being overweight or obese. In many cases, the ovaries are found to contain many small cysts (hence the name), although these are the result of the condition, and not its cause. It is likely that the main cause is high insulin levels, which then also affect the hormones that control the release of an egg (ovulation) each month and regular menstruation. These effects can result in infertility, weight gain and too much androgen (male sex hormones) being produced, causing excess body hair growth. Women with PCOS are at increased risk of developing type 2 diabetes in later life, although some develop prediabetes or type 2 diabetes as early as their teens.

PCOS is usually diagnosed in young women in their teenage years or twenties. It is easy to understand how the various problems it can cause can be very upsetting at this time of life. Treatments are directed at correcting the hormonal imbalance and encouraging weight loss. In my experience, many women with PCOS find it very difficult to lose weight, and I think this is for a number of reasons. Firstly, it can be because they don't feel very good about themselves, and such low self-esteem is a real barrier to making lifestyle changes; secondly, the effects of PCOS in itself can often lead to depression, which can drive unhealthy 'comfort' eating. Finally, and perhaps most importantly, the high insulin levels actually make it very difficult for people to lose weight, especially if they follow a standard low-fat, high-carbohydrate diet that just stimulates yet more insulin to be produced.

Metformin is a treatment for type 2 diabetes that reduces insulin resistance and can be very effective in restoring regular periods, and a low-glycaemic-index diet (i.e. avoiding highly refined carbohydrates) has also been shown to be beneficial. Individuals who are able to lose weight will often find that their periods return as their hormones re-establish a normal balance. It is therefore important to be aware that fertility can return very quickly after starting metformin or changing diet.

Other conditions related to insulin resistance

Insulin resistance is now recognized to contribute to the development of a whole host of conditions. These include fatty liver, dementia, anxiety, depression, some cancers, gout, osteoarthritis, inflammation, heart disease, stroke, high blood pressure and high cholesterol levels. The bad news is that this means that these conditions are more frequent in people with type 2 diabetes and prediabetes. The really good news, however, is that changes you make to reverse the diabetes disease process will also help to reverse insulin resistance and lead to improvements in some of these other conditions.

CHAPTER 3

The implications of a diagnosis of type 2 diabetes

This chapter is in two parts. In the first part, I will set out some of the immediate health implications of a diagnosis of type 2 diabetes. Whether you already have type 2 diabetes, or have prediabetes, the aim is to ensure that you are fully informed about what having type 2 diabetes can mean for your health in the short term. It is not to alarm you, but to reassure you by explaining why you might have a particular symptom or health problem, and importantly to explain what you can do to minimize the impact of diabetes on your health, both more immediately and in the longer term.

The second part of the chapter will cover the different long-term complications of diabetes. Again, the aim is to provide an explanation of why these complications occur, reassurance that they are not inevitable and information about what you can do to minimize the risk of them occurring.

This chapter is included early in the book, as the information may help you refine some of the changes you want to make, in respect of addressing your diabetes or prediabetes.

The immediate health implications of diabetes

In Chapter 2, we learnt how high glucose levels in the bloodstream cause the typical symptoms of diabetes, such as thirst, excessive urination and blurred vision. We also learnt that many people never experience these symptoms, as they are diagnosed before their glucose levels become high enough to result in them. However, having diabetes or prediabetes can also be associated with a number of other, less marked, symptoms that may have crept up gradually over a number of years. Despite being less obvious, they may still have a significant impact on overall wellbeing and health.

One of the most common symptoms that people describe is an overall feeling of lethargy and lack of energy. Often, this is combined with difficulty concentrating and thinking clearly. People often assume this to be a natural effect of getting older, but one of the biggest changes reported by people who manage to reverse their diabetes is that they have so much more energy, and they can think more clearly. Poor sleep is also common in people with diabetes and can contribute to tiredness and poor concentration. People with high blood glucose levels will often have their sleep disturbed by having to get up and pee several times a night. Nerve pain as a result of diabetes can also interfere with sleep. People who are overweight can develop a condition called sleep apnoea, where excessive fat in the neck causes the breathing passages to be restricted, leading to difficulty breathing, and sometimes stopping breathing altogether for several seconds. Often it is the person's partner who is more aware of this condition, as the person themselves may not fully wake during the night, but the breathing disturbances still disrupt the quality of their sleep, so they wake up feeling very tired. As a result, they can fall asleep easily during the day, and that can further disturb the proper night-time sleep rhythm.

Apart from the effects of poor sleep, concentration can be affected by a number of factors related to diabetes that affect brain function. It has been shown that mild cognitive impairment is more common in people with raised glucose levels, insulin resistance, obesity and unhealthy eating patterns. A common manifestation of cognitive impairment is 'brain fog', where people find it difficult to concentrate or remember things. One of the clearest descriptions of brain fog that I have heard came from Tom Watson, former Member of Parliament in the UK and deputy leader of the Labour Party. In 2019, he told a packed meeting in Parliament about the changes he experienced after losing 60 kg (132 pounds) in weight; apart from the obvious physical benefits, he spoke with great clarity about how his mind was sharper and his memory so much better than when he was heavier and had type 2 diabetes.[4] In his book, *Downsizing*, he describes how he became more focused in meetings, could recall facts and figures without prompting and was much better prepared for speeches and interviews.[5]

With poor energy levels and poor concentration, it is perhaps not surprising that people with prediabetes and type 2 diabetes also experience low mood. It is well established that there is a two-way link between depression and type 2 diabetes. The exact mechanism of this is unknown but it has been demonstrated that depressive mood symptoms are worse when blood glucose levels are higher. There is also some evidence that the changes in the brain in people with depression can potentially increase the risk of developing type 2 diabetes, and that clinical depression is at least twice as common in people with diabetes than without. It has been shown that some diabetes medications can help improve symptoms of depression, while following a very low-carbohydrate diet can help symptoms of depression in a person with type 2 diabetes.

As we progress through this book, we will read a number of stories of people's experiences of living with and reversing diabetes. Some common themes emerge about their general health. As well as problems with cognitive function and mental health, gout and acid reflux feature and are increasingly recognized as conditions that occur in people with type 2 diabetes – and often disappear as the diabetes reverses.

People whose blood glucose reaches high levels can experience symptoms directly as a result of the effect of high glucose on nerve function. These symptoms are different from those caused by the gradual damage done to nerves as a result of many years of having high glucose levels in the blood. In fact, these nerve-function issues can occur very early on, and are sometimes what leads a person to go to their doctor, only then to find out that they have diabetes. Nerve cells appear to be particularly sensitive to changes in glucose levels, and this can cause tingling, typically in the feet, that can sometimes become quite painful. Men can also experience erectile dysfunction as a result of the effect of high glucose on the nerves that open up the blood spaces in the penis to cause an erection. These symptoms generally resolve, as the blood glucose levels improve.

Another effect of a high glucose level is an increased risk and severity of infection. This is particularly common with bladder or genital infections, and results from the presence of glucose in the urine, which is a rich breeding ground for bacteria, and also fungal infections such as thrush. People with diabetes can also find that if they get a skin wound or insect bite, it can take longer to heal and may be more likely to become infected than in people without diabetes. For people with more severe complications of diabetes, affecting nerves and blood supply to the feet, as discussed in more detail in the next section, this can lead to severe foot infections that sometimes affect the underlying bone and can result in amputation.

Prior to the Covid-19 pandemic of 2020, for most people, the greater infection risk was little more than a nuisance they could live with, perhaps requiring an occasional course of antibiotics. That all changed with the advent of Covid-19. Within just a few weeks of the first wave in the spring of that year, it became clear that people with diabetes were significantly more likely to become ill and die as a result of becoming infected with the virus. While people with other health problems such as heart disease fared worse, people with type 2 diabetes without any other additional complications were still nearly twice as likely to die as a result of Covid-19 infection than people without diabetes.

So, while we have long known that people with type 2 diabetes are at increased risk of early death, and that those with specific complications such as foot disease are at particular risk, such deaths usually followed a prolonged period of poor health associated with long-term complications of diabetes. Covid-19 was different. Covid-19 caused often rapid death in people who had diabetes but who were otherwise, apparently, well.

What Covid-19 highlighted was that having diabetes has significant effects on the immune system, weakening its ability to fight the infection. This effect proved greatest in those with higher blood glucose levels and those who were overweight. In fact, having a fasting glucose above 7 mmol/l (126 mg/dl) was associated with increased risk of death, even in those who were not known to have diabetes (many such individuals very likely had prediabetes). Much research has been done to identify the many ways in which diabetes has these effects on the immune system:

- High glucose levels increase replication of the SARS-CoV-2 virus responsible for Covid-19, meaning that very quickly the individual is infected with many more virus particles.
- High glucose levels also reduce the effect of killer cells, special immune cells that attack viruses.
- Insulin resistance (seen in overweight people even if they do not have prediabetes or type 2 diabetes) and high glucose levels activate the immune system to cause a state of chronic inflammation, which can cause damage to different tissues in the body.
- Experiments in diabetic mice showed that infection with MERS-CoV (a similar coronavirus) triggers the immune system to cause extensive lung damage, as is seen in people with severe Covid-19 infection.
- Covid-19 infection in people with diabetes increases insulin resistance, causing glucose levels to rise even more and exacerbating these effects.

These effects are not just confined to coronaviruses and we have known for a long time that people with diabetes have an impaired immune system that makes them at increased risk from infections. However, Covid-19 has really highlighted that this increased infection risk is not just a nuisance, it is a potentially deadly consequence of having type 2 diabetes.[6] That is the bad news. The really good news is that the two biggest risk factors – having high glucose levels and being overweight – can both be addressed. In the following chapters, we will explain how prediabetes and type 2 diabetes can be reversed, which will help restore normal functioning of the immune system and protect from Covid-19 and other infections.

The long-term complications of diabetes

The term 'complications of diabetes' generally refers to the long-term effects that diabetes has on various parts of the body. At their worst, these can lead to blindness, kidney failure and amputations. It is a sad fact that many people will have experience of relatives and friends with diabetes who have been affected in this way. Others will have heard (well-meaning) friends tell of the person they know who has become blind and lost both legs as a result of diabetes. On hearing such stories, it is understandable and tempting for someone recently diagnosed with diabetes to become overly fatalistic about the future and not try to control diabetes on the mistaken assumption that significant complications are all but inevitable.

If we go back to the 1970s, it was generally believed that these complications were indeed inevitable: when I was a young doctor in the 1990s, I was told by a much older colleague (although probably younger than I am now!) that, when he was training, his boss told him that you only complete your training in diabetes when a person you diagnose with diabetes loses their eyesight many years later. Quite a horrendous milestone for the patient and an ominous one for the doctor. This was on the basis that it was believed that type 2 diabetes was a progressive condition and that complications such as blindness were inevitable, and there was not much that could be done to stop them.

Nevertheless, even before we learnt that type 2 diabetes can be reversed, we learnt that serious complications are by no means inevitable – especially for someone who is newly diagnosed. In fact, with good management, it is safe to say that the more severe complications can be avoided altogether, and milder ones that might occur can be treated or controlled, ensuring that they do not cause any problems. This is because the risk of complications is directly related to the level of glucose in the bloodstream, usually assessed by the HbA1c blood test (please refer to page 20). Simply put, the higher the HbA1c, the greater the risk of developing complications. Keeping glucose levels as normal as possible (equivalent to an HbA1c between 40 and 50 mmol/mol – roughly 6 to 7 per cent) greatly minimizes the risk of complications. Achieving remission reduces the risk still further; indeed, we are now hearing of cases where things that were once thought of as permanent complications have been reversed as people have reversed their diabetes.

The foundation of good management of prediabetes or type 2 diabetes is making lifestyle changes, right from the time of diagnosis. It is why I consider it so vitally important that at diagnosis people have the opportunity to learn how to best manage their diabetes. There is good evidence that the gains made in the early days and weeks after diagnosis lead to lasting health benefits. In the past, it was not unusual for people to have type 2 diabetes for many years before they were diagnosed, perhaps because the symptoms were initially quite mild or they did not feel unwell enough to visit their doctor. As a result, people could already have evidence of advanced complications of diabetes by the time they were diagnosed. Fortunately, in the UK, this is becoming increasingly rare as more people are aware of diabetes, and GPs and other health professionals have become very good at testing people who are at risk of developing it. In other parts of the world, however, it is a sad fact that people are still often not diagnosed until complications have set in.

If you have recently been diagnosed with prediabetes or type 2 diabetes, I very much hope that, if you follow the advice in this book, you will not experience the complications I am about to describe. Nevertheless, I do believe you need to be aware of them, so that you understand the importance of having the various checks for evidence of complications done on a regular basis, as part of your overall diabetes care. I also want to emphasize the measures that can be taken, both by you as someone with diabetes and by your doctor, to prevent them.

As I have already stated, complications arise as a result of the effect of high blood glucose levels on the body. It is estimated that it takes at least ten years for advanced complications to become established, and so a few weeks or months of high glucose levels are unlikely to lead to lasting damage. The risk of complications is greatest in the cases where glucose levels have been high for years. And whereas type 2 diabetes was originally seen mainly as a 'sugar disease', we now know that high blood pressure and high cholesterol levels are also associated with the development of complications. As people with diabetes tend to have higher blood pressure and cholesterol levels than people without diabetes, ensuring that these are also under good control is as important as managing blood glucose levels.

Vascular disease: damage to large blood vessels

Most of the complications of diabetes are due to damage to blood vessels, known as vascular disease. Blood vessels are commonly divided into large and small blood vessels. Large blood vessels are the tubes that carry blood from the heart to all parts of the body (the arteries) and back from the various parts of the body to the heart (the veins). The heart pumps constantly to maintain blood pressure and to keep blood flowing through the system. As the arteries reach out across the body they divide into smaller and smaller branches until they form very small blood vessels called capillaries. It is here that the nutrients contained within the blood (such as oxygen and glucose) leave the blood vessels and enter the surrounding tissues, where they are used as energy by the cells within the tissue (for example, a muscle). It is a bit like a domestic central heating system: the heart is like the boiler (creating the pressure); the blood vessels are like the copper pipes (carrying the hot water around); and the capillaries are a bit like the radiators (where the energy is transferred to heat the air). However, the analogy then begins to break down as, in the body, capillaries also collect waste products such as carbon dioxide from the tissues to be recycled. Household radiators don't do that, yet.

Just as the pipes in the central heating system can get furred up, leaky or blocked, so can the blood vessels. When we are born, our blood vessels are beautifully smooth and clean inside, but as we grow older the insides of our blood vessels start to fur up with atheroma, so-called narrowing of the arteries. If the narrowing becomes critical, then the part of the body supplied by that blood vessel will be deprived of oxygen and other essential nutrients. At the point when a blood vessel becomes completely blocked, the tissue it supplies will be damaged, and part of it may die to be replaced by scar tissue. If this occurs in a coronary artery in the heart, it is referred to as a heart attack; in the brain, it is called a stroke. Blockage of an artery in the leg may lead to tissue damage in the foot. The underlying process is the same, but the effect depends on which artery is affected and what part of the body it serves.

You will be aware that heart attacks and strokes occur not only in people with diabetes and are actually quite common in our society. There are a number of factors that are associated with an increased risk of these sorts of serious health problems, including smoking, having a family history of such diseases, having high blood pressure or high cholesterol levels and being overweight. Type 2 diabetes is described by some doctors as being part of the 'metabolic syndrome'. This is a group of conditions that are often found together, including diabetes, obesity, high blood pressure and high cholesterol levels. There is evidence that insulin resistance and high insulin levels directly lead to high blood pressure and cholesterol levels, and it is quite possible that this is the main problem in the metabolic syndrome.

Now, there is not much you can do about your family history and if you have high blood pressure or high cholesterol this may also be partly due to the genes you have inherited from your parents. However, everyone can try to stop smoking and lose some weight; indeed, making lifestyle changes that help you lose weight will also reduce your insulin levels and help reduce blood pressure and cholesterol levels. Medications are also available to reduce these where necessary (see Chapter 16). Taken together, such measures can significantly reduce the risk of vascular disease, even in people with diabetes.

Whereas large blood vessel diseases can occur in people without diabetes, small blood vessel disease is more specific to diabetes. This is because it generally results directly from the excess of glucose in the bloodstream. Over time, this excess causes small blood vessels – the capillaries – to become blocked or leaky. While this process will occur to some extent all over the body, its main effects are seen in two critical areas: the eyes and the kidneys.

Diabetic eye disease – retinopathy

Diabetic eye disease (known as retinopathy) is probably the most common complication of diabetes, and also the most studied. This is because it is possible to see directly the damage to the blood vessels in the eye, and document it. Indeed, annual screening for diabetic retinopathy is done by taking a digital image of the back of the eye. Next time you attend for retinal screening, ask the person performing the test to show you the pictures. You will see the retina – the lining of cells inside the back of the eye, which is orange in colour. Just off-centre is a paler circular area (called the optic disc), from which the capillaries fan out to supply blood to all parts of the retina. These are seen as smooth, fine red lines. After many years of high glucose levels, these capillaries can become irregular (leaving tiny red dots poking through the surface) or begin to leak (leaving red or white blots). This is called background diabetic retinopathy and does not affect eyesight. Over time, however, damage to a capillary can cause the area of retina it serves to be starved of oxygen and glucose, and this can change the appearance of the retina. This stage, known as pre-proliferative retinopathy, does not adversely affect eyesight either.

There are two types of retinopathy that do affect vision. The first is a progression of the process described above, where the damaged retina sends out signals to stimulate the formation of new blood vessels to supply the area covered by the defective capillary. This may seem like a good thing, but unfortunately these new capillaries have a tendency to grow forwards into the vitreous (the jelly which fills the eyeball) and they are also very fragile, which means they have a tendency to bleed into the eyeball, and it is this that can cause blindness.

The other type of sight-threatening retinopathy is maculopathy. This is where the retinopathy affects the central part of the retina, the macula. As this area is used for central vision, any damage affects your ability to focus on what you are looking at. This will make it difficult to read, or drive a car, for example, even though the surrounding areas of retina may be relatively unaffected.

As retinopathy can become quite advanced before it notably affects the sight, it is essential that everyone with diabetes has regular screening for retinopathy. This entails having a photograph taken of the back of the eyes (usually once a year) using a camera that looks through the pupil. In the UK, screening is often provided by high-street optometrists or by mobile units that run screening sessions at different locations. It is free of charge. In other countries, screening is done by eye specialists. The good news is that if retinopathy is picked up early, then treatment is available to stop it progressing to the stage where it can affect vision. Laser therapy is the traditional form of treatment; a fine laser beam is shone through the pupil to the areas of retina affected and works by stopping the damaged retina producing the chemical signals that lead to the formation of new blood vessels. It can also help shrink any blood vessels that have already formed and is very effective in preventing blindness. In the past ten years, drug treatments have become available to treat sight-threatening retinopathy. These are given by injection through the front of the eye into the macula and are a class of drugs known as anti-VEGF (vascular endothelial growth factor); they can be very effective in protecting vision, particularly when the macula is swollen (macular oedema).

The other piece of good news is that retinopathy can be prevented by maintaining good control of diabetes and blood pressure, and by stopping smoking. While very mild background retinopathy is not that uncommon in people with longstanding diabetes, sight-threatening retinopathy is almost unheard of in people whose diabetes is well controlled. Further useful information on retinopathy is available at the UK retinopathy screening service website.[7]

Diabetic kidney disease – nephropathy

The other part of the body that is particularly affected by small vessel disease is the kidneys. The kidneys are the essential organs that help maintain the correct balance of chemicals, salts and water in the bloodstream. As the heart pumps blood around the body it passes through the kidneys that sit on either side of the back, just below the ribs. Whereas in most parts of the body, capillaries transfer nutrients to the surrounding cells, the reverse occurs in the kidneys. Here, specialized capillaries transfer waste products into tiny tubes called collecting ducts. These then lead into the ureter, which takes the waste (urine) into the bladder.

Let's take glucose as an example: when the level of glucose in the bloodstream rises above about 10 mmol/l (180 mg/dl), the kidneys try to get rid of the excess glucose by removing it into the urine. This glucose has to be dissolved in water, so the kidneys release extra water into the urine. This naturally results in making the individual pass more urine, leading to dehydration, which in turn causes an obvious thirst and an urge to drink more fluid in an attempt to keep well hydrated. This means that the common symptoms of high glucose levels, namely excess thirst and urination, are the result of the kidneys doing their job in trying to restore more normal levels of glucose in the blood.

The kidneys act a bit like a filter or a fine sieve, allowing only certain things through and into the urine. When the capillaries in the kidney become damaged, the filter becomes leaky (or the holes in the sieve become larger) and this allows substances (such as proteins), which normally should be kept in the bloodstream, to leak out into the urine. Finding the presence of protein in the urine can be a sign that the kidneys have been affected by diabetes.

Just leaking a little extra protein into the urine is itself of little consequence. However, over time, diabetic kidney disease can cause the pressure within the kidneys to rise, which can increase their leakiness. Kidneys are also important in controlling blood pressure, and damage to them can cause the blood pressure to rise, which in turn can increase the pressure in the kidneys, so causing additional damage. Eventually, the kidneys can become seriously damaged and even scarred, making them ineffective in maintaining the correct composition of the blood. This eventually leads to kidney failure and the need for dialysis or a kidney transplant.

Fortunately, just as with diabetic eye disease, this severe form of kidney disease is increasingly rare, and with good care, kidney disease can be prevented. The message is the same and worth repeating: keeping good control of diabetes and blood pressure will avoid these problems. It is important to have a urine test once a year to check if there is the earliest sign of protein leaking into the urine, and if there is, treatments are now available which can help reverse this leak and keep the kidneys healthy. Even people whose kidney function has been moderately affected by diabetes can lead long and active lives thanks to treatments that control blood pressure and prevent any further damage. The most common of such treatments is a class of drugs called ACE inhibitors (such as ramipril or lisinopril, for example). They work by reducing the pressure within the kidneys and as a result can reduce the leak of protein into the urine, helping maintain good kidney function.

Diabetic nerve disease – neuropathy

If the blood vessels are a bit like the heating system in your house, the nerves are analogous to the electrical wiring, providing information (sensation) from all parts of the body and power to all the muscles of the body. Nerves are specialized cells whose function is to transmit tiny electrical currents from one end to the other, so they do act a bit like electrical wires.

Sensory nerves have specialized endings in the tissues that pick up a particular sensation. If, for example, you step on a sharp object such as a pin, nerve endings in the skin will transmit the pain sensation up your leg, up and along the spinal cord to the brain. While the pain itself is unpleasant, it is in fact acting as a protective mechanism for the foot. Within the brain, nerves will connect to the area that controls speech, so that you may well shout 'ouch' or something rather less polite. They will also connect to motor nerves that travel back down the spinal cord, and to the muscles in your leg that now contract quickly to lift your foot away from the painful object. Sensory and motor nerves control almost all functions in the body – from the beating of the heart to the movement of the gut, sweating, sexual function, emptying the bladder and just about everything else.

In diabetes, nerve function can be affected by high glucose levels, both in the short term and in the longer term. The short-term effects can be likened to a toxic effect of glucose on the nerves, and it is not unusual for people to describe a tingling in the feet, or the difficulty of getting an erection during periods when their glucose levels are high – and for these symptoms to improve once the glucose levels stabilize. In the longer term, more permanent nerve damage can occur as a result of high glucose levels. There are a number of possible mechanisms for this and it is likely that the accumulation of glucose within the nerves causes direct damage, as well as nerves being affected by damage to the small blood vessels that supply them.

The longest nerves tend to be affected first, and in most people these are the nerves to the feet, followed by those to the hands. As a result, the most well-known type of neuropathy is that which affects the sensory nerves in the feet. This can lead to tingling and gradually to loss of sensation, so that the feet become essentially numb. The risk here is that stepping on a sharp object simply won't be registered as pain, and this, in turn, may lead to an injury to the foot being left untended. Infection may then set in and might lead to ulceration and more extensive damage to the whole foot. If there is also large vessel disease affecting circulation, then such injuries can be very difficult to heal, and it is this combination that can, in some cases, lead to a need for amputation.

While loss of sensation is perhaps the most common nerve problem in diabetes, the opposite can also occur, where the nerve endings become overstimulated to cause unpleasant tingling or painful sensations. In some cases, these can be improved by good glucose control, but often sufferers need to take medication to reduce the unpleasant sensations.

There are no treatments that can effectively delay or reverse nerve damage and so, as with other types of complication, the key is to prevent it in the first place – by maintaining good control of blood glucose levels. It is important to have your feet examined at least once a year, and more frequently if there is any sign of nerve damage. Hopefully, there will never be any problems, but at the first sign of any sensory problems, it is vitally important to take very great care of your feet in order to minimize any more extensive damage.

Since nerves supply every part of the body, many different bodily functions can be affected by diabetic nerve damage. One of the most common is for men to find it difficult to get an erection. Treatments such as Viagra can be very helpful. More extensive disease can also affect: the sweat glands, causing excessive sweating; the bladder, causing frequent urination or difficulty in passing water; and the gut, causing problems such as heartburn, diarrhoea or constipation. Specific treatments are available that can help control the symptoms of these problems, but they rarely abolish them completely.

Discussion about the long-term complications of diabetes is not easy as, to be frank, they are not very pleasant. However, I do believe it is essential that everyone with diabetes and prediabetes knows about them, as appropriate lifestyle changes early on can greatly help achieve good control of glucose levels and that is the key to preventing them ever occurring in the first place. It is also essential that people with diabetes have the regular check-ups that are designed to detect the earliest signs of any of these problems – so that they can be treated and, in some cases, even reversed. This will be discussed in more detail in Chapter 16. But, above all, it is important to set these complications into context, to be aware that great advances have been made in our ability to prevent them and to treat them.

Even more exciting is the evidence that we are beginning to see in people who have reversed their diabetes already – or even who have only partially reversed it. In Chapter 5, I will describe my experiences helping people reverse their diabetes in Bermuda. One of the great outcomes was how many people achieved much better control of their diabetes, which enabled them to stop their medication. But it was not just diabetes medication they stopped.

A number of people were also able to stop blood pressure medication and others stopped medication for heartburn or painkillers for painful feet. One person remarked, 'My feet feel normal for the first time in years.' And a number of men were delighted to realize that they could manage to perform in the bedroom without the need for Viagra!

As I said earlier, as we progress through the book, I will include a series of real-life stories – first-hand accounts from people who have used some of the principles I recommend. The first is from Steve, who is a retired welder and blacksmith. He lives in the Lake District in north-west England. Here is his story.

STEVE'S STORY

I have always been very fit and active, enjoying cycling, walking and, when I was younger, weightlifting. Despite this, I put on weight as the years went by and found it difficult to keep up with my wife when we walked in the hills. In 2005 at the age of 50, I was diagnosed with type 2 diabetes. When I was diagnosed, I was advised to avoid sugar but otherwise provided with no specific dietary advice. I was started on metformin, and then gliclazide, and after a while started on insulin, ending up on over 80 units a day.

In 2016, my eye screening showed I had some diabetic eye disease. This progressed to the extent that I was advised I would likely need injections into the eye to prevent it deteriorating and affecting my sight. However, soon after, I saw an advertisement in the local newspaper about a course that was being run to help people reverse their diabetes. I showed it to my wife who said I should go. I didn't want to, but went along to see what it was about.

It was run by a man called Eddy who had reversed his diabetes (see Chapter 18), and he explained that if we cut the carbohydrates from our diet, it could help us too. At that time, I weighed 111 kg (245 pounds) and my HbA1c was 97 (11 per cent), despite all the medication I was taking.

I went home with his diet sheet and thought I would give it a go. I cut out potatoes, bread and cereals and lost 2 kg (4 pounds) in the first week. So I continued and lost more weight. We met as a group for 16 weeks and we all got on really well. A sort of competition developed between us as to who could lose the most weight. I continued to cut out carbs and also stopped eating breakfast on most days. The one food that I really missed was porridge, but as I was doing so well with losing weight, I've managed to stay off it ever since.

At the end of the 16 weeks, I weighed 89 kg (196 pounds). I had lost 22 kg (48 pounds) overall and felt fantastic! My HbA1c had come down to 43 (6.1 per cent), despite taking less than half the amount of insulin. I felt so much better, I could walk further and faster and could keep up with my wife on the hills. I also noticed that people were no longer laughing at the sight of me on my bike.

A few weeks later I went back to see the eye specialist, anticipating that I might need injections as she had explained previously. But when she examined my eyes, they were perfectly clear, with no sign of diabetic eye disease and therefore no need for injections. She was amazed and so was I.

PART TWO

Busting
the myths

CHAPTER 4

Diabetes is not your fault

Myth: You have diabetes because you are lazy and eat too much.
Fact: Type 2 diabetes is rising across the world as lifestyles adapt to changing environments.

Do you ever feel ashamed that you developed diabetes or prediabetes? Do you blame yourself? Has anyone implied that it is your fault? It is not. That is a myth.

When I worked at the International Diabetes Federation (IDF), one of my tasks was to oversee the production of the 'IDF Diabetes Atlas'. This is a resource that is published every two years and that estimates the prevalence of diabetes across the globe. It tells an interesting story, or rather a number of interesting stories. The main headline in the most recent (2019) edition is that over 463 million people worldwide are estimated to be living with diabetes.[8] Well over 90 per cent of those are estimated to have type 2 diabetes, and across the globe, about half do not yet know that they have it. And that is without beginning to count all of those with prediabetes, who are likely to number much more. Studies have estimated that up to one in three adults in China have prediabetes. The estimate in the US is that half of all adults have prediabetes.

Note that these are all estimates, based on studies collected from different parts of the world and at different time points. Some countries have no reliable data on numbers of people with prediabetes or type 2 diabetes and so estimates are based on similar countries that do have data. The real number could be lower or higher, but the estimates are the best we have. In 2016, the World Health Organization (WHO) used a different method to calculate its own estimates. It estimated that 422 million people had diabetes, remarkably similar to the IDF estimate in 2015 of 415 million. The bottom line is that type 2 diabetes and prediabetes are now very common conditions in just about every country in the world.

The first 'IDF Diabetes Atlas' was produced in 2000, when it estimated that 151 million people had diabetes. That means that, over 20 years, the number of people with diabetes increased three-fold; over the same time period, the global population increased by about 28 per cent, from 6.1 million in 2000 to 7.8 million in 2020. In other words, if the rate of diabetes increased as a result of the increase in the world population, we would expect the current prevalence to be 193 million – not 463 million. That means 270 million more people developed diabetes than would be expected, and nearly 250 million of those are likely to have developed type 2 diabetes.

So that poses an obvious question: how has this come about? What are the possibilities? Could this be the result of some infection? Could it be the result of a new genetic disease? Or could it be the result of something else?

We can quite readily discount the first two. As we have seen with Covid-19, a disease that spreads by infection usually spreads quite rapidly – in the case of Covid-19, over 100 million developed the disease in the first year, and if left unchecked, it would have spread exponentially over subsequent years. By contrast, genetic changes take several generations to show their impact, and the diseases that result increase much more slowly. The only possible explanation for this rise in prediabetes and type 2 diabetes is that individuals have been affected by something else, most likely something else in their lives that has affected their metabolism.

Changing environments change our lifestyles

So that poses the next question: what has changed in our lives in the past few decades? To help answer this, have a think about everyday life now compared with when you were a child. What has changed about how we live our lives, how we get about, how we communicate with each other, and how we work, play and go shopping? Even if you are only 30 years old, you will be able to remember a time before smartphones, before Facebook, online shopping and online banking. If you are 60 years old, you will remember a time before fast-food restaurants and coffee shops appeared on every high street, before freezers and microwaves appeared in the home, before ready meals and takeaways, and when a can of cola or a packet of crisps was a special treat. You will also remember when most families had one car – or none – and when many more jobs involved manual and physical work. If you are 80 years old, you will remember food rationing after the war, and if you are older than that you may remember food shortages and hunger.

The net effect of all of these changes is that progressively our physical activity levels have reduced; we now spend many more hours sitting down motionless (apart from using our hands on a smartphone, computer keyboard or mouse) than any previous generation in history. Just 25 years ago online shopping was unheard of and purchasing nearly always required travelling to a shopping centre and walking through several shops until you found what you were looking for. Amazon did not exist as a company until 1994 and first arrived in the UK in 1998 as a bookseller. Online banking started in the UK in 1997; until then, many transactions that you can now do at home, or via your phone, required a visit to a bank branch. That year, only 7 per cent of UK households, and 21 per cent of US households, had access to the internet. Arguably, the universal reach of the internet has had a greater effect on our lifestyle than any other innovation since the advent of the motor car.

Although cars have been around since the early 1900s, they were the preserve of the rich until much more recently. In 1970, there were fewer than 10 million cars in the UK but by 2020 there were well over 30 million. In that period, the population grew by just over 20 per cent. So, while in the 1970s many families had no car, multiple-car households are now common. Indeed, for some it has become a rite of passage for teenagers to acquire their own car once they are old enough to drive, and for a family of four living in the same household each to have their own car. And that means no one has to walk or cycle, or take the bus, to get anywhere. I bought my first car when I was 21 after which I cycled and walked much less.

Then there are more subtle differences. Until the 1980s, TVs did not generally have remote controls. If you wanted to switch on your TV, or to switch between one of the three available channels, you had to get up and walk over to the TV set. In 2012, when I started writing the forerunner to this book, *Reverse Your Diabetes*, if you wanted to watch a film at home, you had to go to a high-street shop, rent a DVD, take it home, load a DVD into a player and watch. When the film finished, you had to walk back to the DVD player, remove the DVD and take it back to the rental shop. There was a company called Netflix that would post the DVD out to you, but it wasn't until 2012 that it began its streaming service in the UK, although for many people, their internet speed did not allow streaming of films. Now, in many countries, you can browse, choose and watch a film (or several films) without leaving your sofa. Why is that relevant? Well, as we will learn in Chapter 9, long periods of sitting down are strongly associated with developing prediabetes and type 2 diabetes.

The other major change to our lives has been to our diet. Imagine living in a household that had neither a freezer, nor a microwave. What would that mean for the type of food eaten? It would mean no ice cream or frozen ready meals on demand. It would mean that microwave ready meals did not exist. Of course, nowadays you can buy good-quality 'home-made' ready meals, but the vast majority are likely to be highly processed and refined, and therefore unhealthy. In our imaginary home, meals were much more likely to be prepared from fresh ingredients each day. Up until the 1970s, this wasn't imaginary, it was the reality. Also in the 1970s, fast food was a strange American phenomenon, rarely found in Europe. I have written before about how I remember visiting the first branch of McDonald's to open in the UK in the late 1970s. I was with a friend who was indignant that there were no knives and forks. 'It won't last long,' he said!

I cringe now when I think about it, but when my daughters were young in the late 1990s, we would take them to McDonald's as a treat, or when we couldn't be bothered to cook, sometimes a bit more frequently than I care to remember. And enticed by a 'free' toy, we bought a Happy Meal that, alongside ultra-processed meat and carbohydrate, came with a huge portion of sugar in the form of a soft drink or 'milkshake'.

Up until then, a can of fizzy drink was a special treat, and returning to when I was young, enjoyed very occasionally. The same was true for a packet of crisps. Nowadays, 'Happy Meals' for adults are available everywhere. Okay, they don't come with a toy, but they are called a 'meal deal' and typically include a large bottle of fizzy drink, a sandwich and a packet of crisps. They are bundled together at a good price to entice you to spend a bit extra, and to buy something that you probably don't need. The result is that what just a couple of generations ago was an occasional treat has now become part of many people's everyday diet. And while most people will be aware that a sugary drink is probably not very healthy, many will consider that the sandwich and the snack are probably okay – at least they aren't full of sugar. But as we will see later on, such foods are far from healthy.

Finally, our physical environment can aggravate the effect of other changes to our lifestyle, especially for people who live in a 'food desert'. This is a term to describe areas, often in poorer neighbourhoods, where there are no shops that sell healthy foods. I am lucky enough to live in a small town that has one main shopping street. Along the street are a number of shops selling good-quality fresh foods – including a butcher, greengrocer and baker, as well as two small supermarkets, all within about a 15-minute walk from my home. A few miles down the road are small villages that either have no shops, or just one 'convenience store', which is great if you want to buy tobacco, alcohol or sweet or processed foods, but not so great if you want fresh produce. They are not connected by any bus services so the only options are to eat what is available at the local shop or drive to the nearest town where you can buy fresh food. More recently, there is the option of ordering online, but that usually comes with a delivery charge that might be unaffordable for some people. People who live in a large inner-city or suburban housing estate in a deprived area with no access to a car really *do* have to rely on what is available at the nearest shop. Paradoxically, while fresh food is hard to find in such places, fast-food outlets are often very common, offering a range of highly processed, unhealthy, inexpensive and accessible foods. Unfortunately, many people in poorer (and not so poor) areas in the UK now rely on food banks for donations of food. And sadly, the majority of foods available at food banks, of necessity, are tins and packets of food. Tinned fish and vegetables can be highly nutritious, but scan down the list of foods available and you will see that many are highly processed and less healthy. Fresh food is rarely, if ever, available. Your environment determines what you can eat.

I saw a very nice example of that when I was visiting my colleague, Dr Daniel Katambo, in Nairobi, Kenya. One morning I was sitting at a breakfast table on the terrace of our hotel, enjoying the Africa sun. As is usually the case, on each table was a dish with small packets of sugar to use in your tea or coffee (they like their tea very sweet and very milky by the way). Just ahead of me, a small bird landed on the next table, scooped up a packet of sugar and took off with it. The bird landed on a wire fence a couple of metres away, pecked open the packet and started to eat the sugar inside. One of its friends then came and landed next to it and they proceeded to share the sugar between them. Now, I am sure that birds did not evolve to live off highly refined sugar. But this particular bird was living in an environment where it had a readily available supply of sugar all around and it did not have to go foraging for more traditional (and healthier) food sources.

Our environment can also impact on our activity levels. 'Walkability' is a term used to describe how easy it is to walk in a particular environment, typically a town or city. This is less of an issue in the UK, but in the US, many cities are built with the needs of the car as a priority. Many main roads were built without any pavement (or 'sidewalk' in the US) to allow people to walk safely along them. Walkability can also be affected by perceived danger from attack, especially at night. The provision of cycle lanes also makes a big difference. I am a keen, albeit fair-weather, cyclist and when I lived in Belgium, it was apparent that just about every road had a proper, dedicated cycle path, for cyclists only. Not a narrow strip of the main road where you have to navigate around parked cars, or that disappears every so often, or moves onto the pavement (sidewalk) because the road is too narrow. The huge increase in cycling in London over the past 20 years has been a great success and to the benefit of many people's health. However, the narrow roads and lack of cycle lanes has also led to far too many injuries and deaths arising from collisions with large vehicles. If people feel safe, they are more likely to cycle; if not, they will use their car.

The effect of changing lifestyles on obesity and type 2 diabetes

These examples are to illustrate how our lifestyles have changed very significantly over the past few decades. These changes are largely because of changes to our environment – whether it is our food environment, technological environment or our physical environment. That in itself need not be a bad thing. However, alongside these changes in lifestyle, we have witnessed significant adverse changes in our health. Obesity rates have risen steadily since the 1990s in adults, and more alarmingly, in children. By the age of 11, around one in three children in the UK is over-weight or obese. And two in three adults are now overweight or obese.

Obesity is diagnosed by calculating an individual's body mass index (BMI). This is the relationship between a person's height and their weight. Normal body weight is defined as a BMI between 20 and 25. A BMI between 25 and 30 is defined as overweight, and one above 30 as obese. The precise calculation is to take the weight in kilograms and to divide it by the square of the height in metres. Thus, for a person who weighs 80 kg (about 176 pounds) and is 1.83 m tall (about 6 feet), the BMI is calculated as:

$$80/(1.83 \times 1.83) = 23.9 \text{ (which would be in the normal range)}$$

A person of the same height who weighs 110 kg (about 242 pounds) has a BMI of $110/(1.83 \times 1.83) = 32.9$ (which is in the obese range). A chart to help work out your BMI is in Appendix B.

The BMI is generally not used for children and care must be taken with individuals who are very muscular. Muscle weighs more than fat, and it is quite possible for someone to be 'overweight' but actually be very fit and healthy, with an increased body weight because of large muscles. It has been suggested that waist circumference is a better measure of obesity as most people who are genuinely overweight owing to fat have large fat stores around their middle.

Until the 1990s, type 2 diabetes was not readily associated with obesity. Certainly there were people who were obese and had type 2 diabetes, but there were also many people with type 2 diabetes who, while a little overweight, were not obese at diagnosis.

I know this because, at the hospital where I worked, an education programme for people newly diagnosed with type 2 diabetes was started in 1993. Everybody who was diagnosed by their GP was referred to the diabetes centre within a week of the diagnosis so they might attend education sessions over the following weeks.

At the first session everyone was weighed, and detailed records were kept on everyone who presented with new-onset type 2 diabetes until the programme transferred out of our centre in 2005. In 1995, there were thought to be about 1 million people in the UK with type 2 diabetes. During that year, 367 people newly diagnosed with type 2 diabetes were referred to our education programme. Their average body weight was 82 kg (181 pounds) with a BMI of 29, which is in the overweight range.

What happened over the next ten years was striking. Firstly, there was a steady increase in the number of people diagnosed with type 2 diabetes, so that in the year 2000 nearly 800 people attended the programme, and by then the total number of cases in the UK had doubled to 2 million. There had been a slight increase in the average weight of people newly diagnosed with diabetes to 84.5 kg (186 pounds). For the next few years, the numbers with newly diagnosed diabetes continued to increase, as did their weight, and by 2005 the average weight was 89 kg (196 pounds), over 7 kg (or 15 pounds) heavier than their counterparts who had been diagnosed ten years earlier. By then, hardly anyone was of normal body weight. Type 2 diabetes had become a disease of the overweight and obese, much like the very early historical accounts of the disease. And by 2020, there were over 4 million people in the UK with type 2 diabetes – and it is estimated that over 30 per cent of the general population were obese.

This has led to a big shift in the way we think about the disease. In the 1990s, people were reassured that they did not get diabetes as a result of their diet or lifestyle. Rather, their diabetes was due to unknown factors and beyond their control, perhaps in their genes. Yet (and perversely), they were also told that changing their lifestyle would help control it. Thirty years later, with the twin epidemics of diabetes and obesity visited upon us, and the close correlation between the two, it is abundantly clear that – in many cases – diabetes has developed in individuals as a result of them being overweight. And for the number of people developing diabetes to have increased so much in just a few years means it cannot be due to some sort of genetic disposition alone. The message is now very clear: our modern lifestyles mean that many of us have become overweight. And if you become overweight there is a greatly increased chance of developing diabetes. The bad news is that on an individual level this means that there is a direct link between a person's lifestyle and later development of diabetes; the good news is that this readily explains why lifestyle changes can help control diabetes – and raises the exciting possibility that changing lifestyle might help reverse the condition.

Let me just add that, while the majority of people in the UK with type 2 diabetes are overweight, some people are not overweight when they develop diabetes. Remember that type 2 diabetes arises as a result of excess fat in the liver. While, in many cases, this occurs in the presence of more widespread fat excess around the body, i.e. in people who are overweight, some people accumulate sufficient excess fat in their liver to cause type 2 diabetes, even though their BMI could be within the normal range. This is particularly common in people of Asian ethnicity.

This phenomenon of rising cases of type 2 diabetes is not just occurring in rich Western countries. The biggest increases in type 2 diabetes are occurring in countries in Africa and Asia, where urbanization, and the changes associated with it, has been shown to be a key factor in driving it. The tragedy is that these countries lack the resources to be able to identify cases early and provide appropriate treatment; as a result, increasing numbers of people are suffering the consequences of untreated diabetes, leading to premature disability and death.

Learning from the Bermuda Triangle of diabetes

In 2015, I was invited to stop off in Bermuda on my way back from a diabetes conference in the US. I was asked by the Bermuda Diabetes Association to give a presentation about reversal of type 2 diabetes, following the successful publication of my book. All I knew about Bermuda was that it sounded like a nice place to visit and the men there wore shorts. I thought it was near the Caribbean – but even that was wrong, as Bermuda is about 1,400 km (900 miles) further north, about three-quarters of the way across the Atlantic, on about the same latitude as North Carolina. I flew in from Boston on a flight that took about two hours, landing at lunchtime. I gave my talk in the afternoon and then flew out that evening back to London. I was on the island for all of six hours. But it did look very nice.

I thought nothing more of it, but a few months later I was contacted by a local Bermudian GP, Dr Stanley James, who said he had read my book and would like to set up a programme, based on the principles within it, essentially recommending a low-carbohydrate diet for people with type 2 diabetes. We kept in contact and, a year later, he asked if I could go out there and set up a programme. It sounded like a great idea, and so my wife and I travelled out to Bermuda for a week towards the end of 2016 on a fact-finding mission and to meet with various stakeholders to seek their support for such an initiative. And to find a beach or two.

Bermuda has an estimated prevalence of diabetes of over 13 per cent, over twice as high as the UK (at 6 per cent) and higher even than the US (10 per cent). And during that week it was easy to see why. Soon after we arrived, we went to a local grocery store to pick up some basics. The first thing we noticed was that most of the produce comes from the US. The second was the huge array of sugary drinks – again, most were from the US, but I did notice the local Bermudian ginger beer with 48 g (about 12 teaspoons) of sugar in one can (by comparison, regular Coca-Cola has 35 g or about 9 teaspoons). And the third thing we noticed was the high cost of everything, particularly the fresh produce. Fruit and vegetables were up to three times more expensive than in the UK. The 'average' wage in Bermuda is at least twice that of the UK, but this is skewed by some very high earners; many people earn a similar amount as in the UK. For low earners, food – and fresh food in particular – is disproportionately expensive.

To get to the store, we had to walk along a narrow road with no pavement. All roads in Bermuda are narrow, shared by cars, trucks and motorcycles, as well as the occasional intrepid pedestrian. Walking one of those roads, especially in the dark, really does make you feel vulnerable.

To avoid over-congestion on the roads, households are limited to one car each; this means that many people use mopeds to get around the island. In fact, adding the total numbers of cars and mopeds gives Bermuda a higher density of private motorized transport than the UK. The great 'advantage' of riding a moped is that you literally can ride door to door, so that if you have a moped (and acquiring one at the age of 16 is common practice) you hardly have to walk anywhere at all.

By the time I met the Minister of Health to discuss setting up a diabetes programme, I had experienced enough in just a couple of days to understand why Bermuda had such a high rate of type 2 diabetes. The food environment provided highly processed and high-sugar produce at low cost compared with the much more expensive healthier options. The densely populated physical environment afforded limited opportunities for walking (unless you were a member of one of the expansive golf clubs), and this, together with the reliance on private motorized transport, meant that walking was just not part of the culture. The combination of unhealthy diet, adverse physical environment and low physical activity together constitute the Bermuda Triangle of diabetes.

Now, before you start wondering if you have picked up the wrong book (why all this stuff about Bermuda, I hear you ask), the reason for including this information is to highlight how what we eat and drink and how we behave are hugely determined by our environments. And as our environments change, so do our behaviours. Bermuda is a group of small volcanic islands, so its geography has changed very little in the past 100 years. However, the use of the land has changed dramatically. Agricultural land has been squeezed out by property developments, walking has been replaced by motorized transport, and home produce replaced by imported food.

As food production around the world has become globalized, there has been a shift towards more highly processed foods, and their successful marketing means that sugar-sweetened drinks are now a significant part of many people's diet. As a result, whole populations have changed their diet and physical activity levels, and many individuals have, as a result, developed type 2 diabetes. It is, therefore, much too simplistic to lay the blame for a person developing type 2 diabetes on that individual. Just as the bird I saw eating sugar in Kenya, and as all human populations in history, we adapt to eat the food in our environments. Unfortunately, and probably for the first time in the history of humankind, that has led directly to widespread ill health among many populations.

The foods that increase the risk of diabetes

In 2014, the medical journal *The Lancet* published a review of the evidence about which foods are associated with an increased risk of developing type 2 diabetes.[9] Note that if a food is associated with an increased risk, it does not mean that the food is the cause of type 2 diabetes, but it warrants looking in more detail to see what effect it could be having. There are other research papers that give slightly different messages, but the same key themes keep coming through, and I suggest we can use these to make some sensible decisions about which foods to recommend, and which to avoid, if we want to reverse prediabetes or type 2 diabetes.

There are strong associations with sugar-sweetened beverages (including fizzy drinks and 'natural' fruit juices) and white rice; there is also evidence that excessive consumption of potatoes, especially chips/French fries, is associated with an increased risk of diabetes. What do all of these foods have in common? They all lead to a rapid increase in the level of glucose in the bloodstream, causing the pancreas to secrete more insulin, and increasing the likelihood of accumulating fat in the liver. There is also interesting evidence that suggests that consuming excess sugar may contribute to the development of diabetes, even in people who are not overweight.

Eating processed red meat and takeaway foods is also associated with an increased risk of type 2 diabetes, whereas a vegetarian or Mediterranean diet (rich in green vegetables and healthy fats such as olive oil, nuts and oily fish) are both associated with reduced risk. It is not clear whether it is the meat per se that increases the risk of type 2 diabetes, or the foods eaten with it (the bun with the burger, for example) – either way there is an association. Our ancestors have eaten red meat for thousands of years, long before type 2 diabetes was a health problem, so it is unlikely that moderate intake of good-quality red meat is in itself inherently harmful. On the other hand, yoghurt, nuts, leafy green vegetables and moderate alcohol consumption are associated with a reduced risk of developing diabetes. I have summarized the findings of *The Lancet* paper in Table 4.

Table 4: Foods associated with a reduced and increased risk of type 2 diabetes

Foods associated with reduced risk of type 2 diabetes	Foods associated with increased risk of type 2 diabetes
Carbohydrates	
Brown rice	White rice
Wholewheat bread	Potatoes
Oats	French fries
Fat	
Nuts	
Peanut butter	
Protein	
Yoghurt	Red meat
Dairy products	Processed meat
Specific foods	
Coffee	Fruit juice

Tea	Sugar-sweetened beverages
Moderate alcohol	Excess alcohol
Green leafy vegetables	
Fruit (up to 3 per day)	
Diets	
Mediterranean diet	Restaurant meals of hamburgers, fried chicken, fried fish and Chinese-style food
Vegan or vegetarian diet	High energy density diet

The consumption of the foods in the right half of Table 4 has increased significantly in the past 20 years and probably goes a long way to explaining why the prevalence of type 2 diabetes has increased so much. Therefore, in an attempt to reverse the changes that have led to prediabetes or type 2 diabetes, it would make sense to cut down on those foods associated with increased risk (sugar, potatoes, fast food, white rice and for that matter other refined carbohydrates such as white bread or pasta) and to increase the intake of leafy green vegetables, nuts and unsweetened yoghurt. We will consider this in more detail in Chapters 6 and 11.

This research begs the question: what would happen if those unhealthy foods were suddenly no longer available? In 2020, there was a 'natural experiment' that gave many of us an experience of a sudden change in food availability. As a result of the coronavirus pandemic, many countries went into lockdown, a word that most people had probably never used before. In the UK, the first lockdown started in March 2020. It was not as strict as in some other countries, but all restaurants were closed, including all fast-food takeaway restaurants that were traditionally open 7 days a week, and in some cases 24 hours a day. In an instant they were all closed. I remember thinking at the time what an incredible opportunity for people to make changes to their diets – for the better. For people who regularly used these restaurants, they would have been forced to change their normal eating pattern. And it gave me the idea of creating a survey to see how this affected people, particularly those with diabetes.

I set up an online survey and used social media contacts to ask people with and without diabetes to complete it. I collected responses from over 250 people, including 96 people with type 2 diabetes from 20 countries across all continents. Not surprisingly, many people reported that during lockdown they were eating more at home and eating more fresh foods and a lot less fast food. Nearly 30 per cent decided to use lockdown to eat more healthily, mainly by reducing their intake of sugar and other carbohydrates. A similar proportion reported that they had lost weight during lockdown and nearly a quarter of those with diabetes said that their glucose control had improved. Conversely, another 30 per cent reported that they had gained weight, and 18 per cent that their glucose control was worse.

Once the restaurants opened up again, there were long tailbacks of cars waiting to be served at the drive-in counters, suggesting many people had gone back to their previous eating habits. However, this did provide an example of how a change to the food environment inevitably leads to a change in eating patterns, with potentially significant effects on health, whether good or bad.

Food addiction

Many people will relate to having favourite foods – ones that they like so much they can't get enough of them. We often use the term 'moreish' to describe them – as in 'these biscuits are so moreish' – which actually means 'I enjoy these biscuits so much I just want more'. For some people, it is cheese; for some, it is bread; for others, it is chocolate, or biscuits, or ice cream. Very rarely do I hear people describe broccoli or spinach as moreish. Now, if we are able to control our intake of our favourite foods, then our liking for them is not a problem. However, increasingly, it is recognized that some people cannot control how much they eat, and they even behave as if they are addicted to certain foods, in much the same way as people can become addicted to alcohol or drugs.

I can certainly relate to this. I find ice cream, especially good-quality ice cream made with real cream, extremely moreish. So much so that, if there is a tub of it sitting in the freezer, I find it very difficult not to eat it. And I have been known to eat a very large amount in one go. Eating ice cream gives me an almost instant feeling of pleasure, much more than the taste itself, that drives me to keep on eating it. In fact, this is one type of food that I try to avoid having in the house on a regular basis, because I know I will eat it. I used to have a similar relationship with milk chocolate, but since I switched to 70 per cent or higher dark chocolate, I find milk chocolate unpleasantly sweet. Despite the excess sweetness, which I recognize as no longer being to my taste, it still has that moreish attraction that would get me going back for more. The other food that has that effect on me is bread. Not highly processed white bead, but real, freshly baked sourdough bread, especially with seeds embedded in the crust. Much healthier than ice cream, but still a carbohydrate that would raise blood glucose levels in a person with diabetes.

Some people report that, not only do they lack control when eating certain foods but also, if they do not have them, they develop cravings for them, to the extent that they would make a specific trip out to buy some, just like a smoker who has run out of cigarettes. Why is this?

A lot of research has looked into the effects of different foods on the brain, and it appears that some have similar effects to addictive substances, such as alcohol or drugs. Sugar, in particular, stimulates the pleasure centres of the brain and leads to the secretion of dopamine, which has a great feel-good effect. These effects are particularly marked with fructose, or fruit sugar. In addition, fructose counteracts the effect of leptin, the hormone that is designed to tell us when we are full and when to stop eating. Fructose also increases the accumulation of fat in the liver, a key step in the development of type 2 diabetes. Added sugar in foods is usually sucrose (table sugar), which is made up of 50 per cent fructose and 50 per cent glucose. Some foods and drinks have high-fructose corn syrup (HFCS) instead, which can be as much as 90 per cent fructose. Therefore, it can be seen that any food with added sugar will encourage you to eat more of it *and* potentially directly increase your risk of developing type 2 diabetes. Sugar has similar properties to alcohol (making you want more and increasing fat in the liver) and there is, I believe, a valid argument for treating sugar in the same way as alcohol, with restrictions on its availability, in order to avoid harm to those who consume it.

The addictive effects of sugar help explain my relationship with ice cream and chocolate. If you remember, I also have trouble controlling the amount of bread I eat. Bread has very little, if any, sugar in it. However, it is high in starch and starch is just sugar molecules joined together that, when we eat them, separate out to become glucose. This process starts as soon as we chew bread (and other starchy foods) in our mouths, thanks to the enzyme amylase in our saliva, and some people can taste the sweetness within a few seconds of chewing. So, it is easy to see that addiction to bread, for example, is a variation on sugar addiction, and the term 'carb addiction' is sometimes used to describe an addiction to starchy foods.

There is evidence that fat has similar but less marked effects. However, the combination of sugar and fat has been found to be particularly effective at stimulating addictive overeating. Where do we find that combination? Yes, you guessed it, in all the most addictive foods, including cakes, biscuits and ice cream. And pizza. Some companies add HFCS to pizza crust to give in that golden brown colour – a cynic would say they also know that adding sugar increases its addictiveness, and makes us want to buy a supersize, which we don't really need.

The food industry exploits the addictiveness of certain ingredients, and manufacturers have developed a real expertise in adjusting the composition of their products, precisely to make us want to eat more. Then they market those products with advertising that is designed to trigger certain feelings that make us want to buy the product.

Dan Parker, who used to market junk food until he developed type 2 diabetes, put it to me like this: 'Advertising food is not about nutrition or health or even taste. It's all about emotions. People eat at McDonald's and drink Coca-Cola because advertising creates strong emotional connections between you and their products. As an example, the "Happy Meal" is designed to associate eating at McDonald's with being happy. One of the most powerful emotions is despair. Despair is the difference between expectation and reality. Despair is the single most powerful component used by advertisers to get people to eat junk food: I've had a bad day therefore I deserve a bucket of ice cream.'

Many people with type 2 diabetes have been told that, unless they eat the 'correct' diet (which has historically recommended they control their glucose levels by eating carbohydrates with every meal), they risk going blind or losing a leg. Yet when they follow the advice they are given, their glucose levels rise and their weight increases, largely because they are eating so much carbohydrate. Sometimes they are made to feel like they are to blame, so they experience fear and criticism, which reinforce the gap between their expectation of where they should be and the reality of where they are. That feeds exactly the despair that advertisers exploit to entice us to indulge in their products, which will further widen that gap of despair.

The title of this chapter is 'Diabetes is not your fault'. It is no coincidence that countries with a high incidence of type 2 diabetes also have a high intake of processed foods, refined carbohydrates and sugar-sweetened beverages, which have been cleverly formulated and relentlessly marketed to change not just the food environment but also, often unconsciously, our purchasing behaviour. It is not that people, over the past few decades, have made a conscious decision to become less healthy or to harm their health deliberately. It is not their (or your) fault!

Thankfully, things are beginning to change. Many countries have now introduced different forms of sugar tax, usually on sugar-sweetened beverages. This was first introduced in Mexico in 2014 and within a short time led to a decrease in consumption of sugar and increased use of plain water. The UK followed suit in 2018 but first the government gave the drinks industry two years' notice, so they had the time to reformulate their products to reduce their sugar content and avoid the tax. That, too, was successful in reducing sugar consumption in drinks – by 12.5 g (about three teaspoons) per person each week.[10]

However, for people who show signs of addiction to certain foods, it can be really difficult to get help. Just knowing that certain foods are unhealthy won't be enough to make them change what they eat. Everyone knows that smoking is bad for our health. Even people who smoke 60 cigarettes a day. That knowledge is often not enough to prompt them to stop smoking, as the cravings and the addictive effects are too strong. Smoking, however, is recognized as being addictive, and bodies such as the WHO have developed major initiatives at a global level to discourage it. Food addiction, by contrast, is not even recognized as a condition. There are a growing number of professionals who have developed expertise in this area, and who are encouraging the WHO to introduce a diagnosis of 'disorder due to harmful use of foods'. If successful, that would mean that people affected would not be told to go away and manage their portion sizes or change the foods they eat but would instead be offered treatment to help them understand how these foods affect their brain and their feelings and to help them start the process of cutting out the food in question. Until then, if you recognize that you might struggle with addiction to certain foods, then just 'cutting down' or 'eating in moderation' is unlikely to work. I encourage you to recognize that you may need help to cut out those foods completely.

Joanne's story shows how, with a little help, she managed to do this. Joanne lives in London with her husband and son. She works from home, providing support for academic researchers, often spending long hours sitting at her desk. This is her story.

JOANNE'S STORY

I was diagnosed with type 2 diabetes in 2020 when I was 61. At the time, my HbA1c was 53 (7 per cent) and I weighed 125 kg (275 pounds). I have been overweight since I was a child and I have never really given much thought to my health, as I was strong physically and did not suffer much illness. I always considered my diet to be varied and healthy, with lots of fruit and vegetables, not too much sweet food and moderate alcohol intake. However, I had been taking medication for high blood pressure for many years and in recent years I was feeling increasingly exhausted, and I gained more weight, even though my diet stayed the same, which made me unhappy.

My GP asked if I wanted bariatric surgery, which I refused immediately. Then he just said it would help if I were to lose weight. At that point, I didn't understand about the effect of carbohydrates, and I said I didn't really eat sweet things. He simply replied that it wasn't just sweet things. I asked if I could resolve things through diet and exercise and he said no, that that sort of thing never works. To quote him directly, 'It's all shakes and things and isn't sustainable.' He sent me away in tears, clutching a prescription for metformin and atorvastatin. I didn't take the medication. Instead, when I got home, I went online and found the Diabetes UK Forum, which helped hugely. I immediately cut down on carbs in all forms, and that has made a massive difference.

I started to keep a food diary as that helped reassure me that my calculations were correct. I stopped having my usual multi-seed toast for breakfast, and started to eat different things, like a small cheese and spinach omelette, or mushrooms, bacon and tomatoes, or sometimes a small mixed plate of things like avocado, walnuts, blueberries and some cheese, in fact anything I fancied that didn't have a high carb impact. I also started eating later in the day, so following the 16:8 'fasting' regime, which I found really easy.

It usually meant that my 'breakfast' lasted until my evening meal. Before I would have probably had some bread for lunch, and bread often figured with the evening meal too. Now if I cook pasta, rice or couscous for my son and husband I have 'cauliflower rice' or just lots of salad or vegetables in place of the carbohydrate with the other elements. I have also discovered, and love, celeriac, as a potato substitute. My husband and son are not bothered, they accept it, and always understand if I change things around a bit. I learnt about these replacements by reading the forum. I am not too strict though and I do have the occasional roast potato as a Sunday treat or literally half a dozen chips with fish.

Within two months, my HbA1c had come down to 46 (6.4 per cent). I haven't found it that hard. The food I really miss is bread as it was always something I considered a treat or a comfort. I eat Burgen bread as it is lower in carbs. And I eat that sparingly but sometimes I really want toast for breakfast. Sometimes the chaps will have lovely thick slices of good-quality bread, and I thought that would bother me, but it doesn't really.

I have been driven by a determination not to have to deal with the worst possible scenarios of diabetes, and if I'm honest the way my GP, and the nurse, dealt with me has made me determined not to have to go on medication. I'm a real person, not just this problem to be medicated and sent away. It is my condition and I must be the expert in it, given the lack of expertise that they displayed. I find it very frustrating that what seems to be such an easy way to help people is being ignored by those who could help so much. If I hadn't 'rebelled' against the medical advice I was given, I would probably be eating the same diet and taking more and more medication just to stay in the same place or worse.

I have more energy, I can now walk further, faster, and without dreading it beforehand. I haven't been weighing myself but know I've lost weight as there's a skirt I wear at home which I now have difficulty keeping up! It has become a symbol, and I know that as long as it's happening, I'm doing okay.

Obviously, nobody wants to have a condition which could have serious consequences. I'm aware that even though my last blood test result said I was in the prediabetic range, the diabetes will always be there, waiting to welcome me back. But it's going to be disappointed. It has made me more conscious of my health, I can't take things for granted. I count that as a good thing.

Looking back, I think my job has contributed to my diabetes. I would be sat down for hours and hours, staring at a computer screen. I am self-employed and if deadlines have been pressing, I have been known not to leave the flat for days on end, just working all hours, stopping to cook and eat the evening meal, then collapsing in front of the TV. I've realized how ridiculously damaging that is, and since my diagnosis have done, please don't laugh, a Mr Motivator YouTube session every day, which are surprisingly good workouts! I also make sure I go out for a walk every day and know that I cannot afford to slip back into old ways as my life literally depends on it.

CHAPTER 5

Prediabetes and type 2 diabetes can be reversed

Myth: Prediabetes leads on to type 2 diabetes, which is an inexorably progressive condition that requires progressively more medication and eventually insulin to control it.

Fact: Both prediabetes and type 2 diabetes can be reversed.

Reversal of prediabetes

In 1998, a landmark study was published called the UK Prospective Diabetes Study.[11] The study followed up many people who were diagnosed with type 2 diabetes in the 1970s and 1980s to see what happened to them over the next 12 years. There were two important messages. The first was that if people were encouraged right at the beginning to make changes to their diet that improved their blood sugar levels, this improvement had a beneficial effect over many years. However, the second message was that over the years, blood glucose levels gradually but definitely increased, even in those who made beneficial changes at the beginning. This led to the understanding that type 2 diabetes is an inevitably progressive disease that over time will just get worse and likely need more and more medication.

It was also believed that many people with prediabetes (then called impaired glucose tolerance) would progress to develop type 2 diabetes, and that there was nothing that could be done to halt that. Indeed, when I worked in the Bournemouth Diabetes Centre, we ran an education programme for people with newly diagnosed type 2 diabetes who were referred by their GP. Occasionally, people with prediabetes would turn up. We used to tell them that they shouldn't have been sent along as they did not have diabetes. However, we told them that they were likely to develop type 2 diabetes at some stage, and when they did, they should come back so that we could give them advice on managing it. That was just over 20 years ago, and I cringe when I think of the ill health that could have been prevented if we knew then that type 2 diabetes was not inevitable, and that we could have advised them to make changes to stop them from developing it.

In the early 2000s, research was published that showed that if people with prediabetes were encouraged to change their lifestyle, then they could reduce the risk of developing type 2 diabetes. The advice given was to follow a low-fat, high-fibre diet (therefore high in wholegrains), to lose weight and to increase physical activity. Although the diet was relatively high in carbohydrates, the overall changes were an improvement on their previous diet and would have entailed a reduction in sugar intake. As a result, the risk of developing type 2 diabetes was significantly reduced.

The first such study was the Diabetes Prevention Program, in the US, which was published in 2002 in the *New England Journal of Medicine*.[12] In this study, people with prediabetes were randomly split into different treatment groups. The first group, called the lifestyle intervention group, received advice from an individual case manager for 16 weeks on how to change their diet and lifestyle with the aim of losing weight. They were specifically advised to follow a low-fat, low-calorie diet and to exercise for 30 minutes at least 5 times a week. The second group received the diabetes drug metformin (which lowers blood glucose by making the body's insulin more effective, see Chapter 13) and the third group received a dummy placebo pill (control group). All participants were followed up for four years, during which time those in the lifestyle intervention group were reviewed every month to check on their progress. The results were striking: in each year of the study, 5 per cent of the lifestyle intervention group developed diabetes compared with 11 per cent in the placebo group. Those taking metformin were somewhere between the two. The researchers then went back to check up on the participants ten years after the beginning of the study, and although the intervention had stopped after four years, the benefits continued with a 43 per cent reduction in diabetes in the lifestyle intervention group compared with the control group.

The other main prevention trial was the Finnish Diabetes Prevention Study, published in 2003.[13] This provided similar advice but less intensively (seven sessions in the first year and then every three months for three years), with exercise sessions provided free of charge to participants. Over three years, 9 per cent of subjects developed diabetes compared with 20 per cent in a control group (who did not receive the same advice). In other words, the lifestyle changes reduced the risk of developing diabetes by over 50 per cent. The very strong message from these studies is that type 2 diabetes can be prevented by losing weight, and that diet and exercise are more effective than medication.

So impressed were we with these data that we set up a pilot study in Bournemouth. People with prediabetes were identified by their GP and invited to attend a programme of four sessions on diet and exercise, followed by monthly review groups. Not only did they then not progress to diabetes, after one year their blood tests (including a glucose tolerance test) had returned to normal. This meant that their prediabetes had been reversed. It was only some years later that I went back to the original research papers to see that in the Diabetes Prevention Program in the US, over 40 per cent of people who underwent lifestyle education had reversed their prediabetes at one year. However, this also occurred in over 20 per cent who were in the placebo group. Now it is worth pointing out that people in this group were provided with information about a healthy diet and so some could have acted on this and made changes, even if they did not receive the full advice and support that the lifestyle intervention group had. However, the fact that so many people reversed their prediabetes challenged the view that prediabetes was part of an irreversible process and showed that some people can move in and out of prediabetes. This is hugely encouraging and emphasizes that, for someone who has been diagnosed with prediabetes, there is everything to play for. It is certainly not inevitable that you will go on to develop diabetes. And for people who are willing to make lifestyle changes, there is a high likelihood of reversing prediabetes and hopefully for good.

It is worth pointing out that the Diabetes Prevention Program study started in the 1990s, when the recommended dietary advice was to follow a low-fat diet. This was reasonably effective – the intervention group lost an average of 6 kg (13 pounds) and 40 per cent reversed their prediabetes after one year. Yet, over the following few years, they regained some weight and after four years only 25 per cent were still in remission. More recently, Dr David Unwin, a GP from the north of England, has published results of the effect of advising a lower-carbohydrate diet in 71 people with prediabetes. After an average of nearly two years, they lost over 8 kg (18 pounds) in weight and a staggering 93 per cent had reversed their prediabetes.

So what do we mean by reversal of prediabetes? As we discussed in Chapter 2, type 2 diabetes develops gradually over a period of years as blood glucose levels increase. It is not an on/off event, and the point at which people develop diabetes is defined by a certain level of blood glucose, or more commonly nowadays by the HbA1c blood test.

To recap, prediabetes occurs in a person when their HbA1c is between 42 and 48 mmol/mol (6.0 and 6.5 per cent), or when their fasting blood glucose is between 6.1 and 7 mmol/l (or 110–125 mg/dl). Although by definition they do not have diabetes, there is usually already evidence of metabolic abnormality with insulin resistance as a result of excess fat in the liver. So, reversal occurs when, as a result of lifestyle change, a person is able to reduce their HbA1c to below 42 mmol/mol or 6.0 per cent, or their fasting glucose to below 6.1 mmol/l (110 mg/dl). Keeping it below these levels for at least three months indicates that prediabetes is in remission.

If you have been diagnosed with prediabetes, then in many ways you are very lucky. Lucky because, although you have been identified as being at risk of type 2 diabetes, you have been picked up sufficiently early to be able to do something about it, and hopefully turn your health around and minimize the risk of ever developing diabetes. This is very different from our understanding of the situation 20 years ago.

Reversal of type 2 diabetes: a journey of discovery

If you have been diagnosed with type 2 diabetes, then the disease process has progressed so that the HbA1c is already above 48 mmol/mol or 6.5 per cent. The progression from 'normal' through 'prediabetes' to 'diabetes' is a continual gradual process, with the definitions of each being arbitrarily set. It is not an on/off situation, like, for example, classical type 1 diabetes or lung cancer – where you either have it or you don't. The interventions described above have shown that it is possible to slow down the progression from prediabetes to diabetes and to reverse it from prediabetes to normal. The next big question is: can the situation be reversed once a person already has type 2 diabetes?

As we have seen, 20 years ago the standard answer to this was no. Type 2 diabetes was seen as a progressive condition that just got worse – not better. It was considered to be irreversible and, once diagnosed, a disease for life. All in all, a rather depressing prospect. However, since then several pieces of research have shown that this is not true. Type 2 diabetes can in fact be reversed.

The first evidence for this came from people with diabetes who were also obese, and who underwent bariatric surgery to treat their obesity. Bariatric surgery describes a number of operations that all have the same aim – limiting the amount of food that can be absorbed through the gut into the bloodstream. There are three common types of surgery undertaken in the UK: laparoscopic (keyhole) adjustable gastric banding, laparoscopic gastric bypass and laparoscopic sleeve gastrectomy. The gastric band is the simplest procedure, whereby an inflatable ring is placed around the top of the stomach in order to reduce the amount of food that can enter the stomach at any one time.

The width of the band is adjusted by injecting water into it to inflate it. Whereas the gastric band can be adjusted or even removed, the sleeve gastrectomy is a permanent operation that achieves the same aim by surgically narrowing the stomach to a thin tube. These procedures have no effect on the rest of the gut. Gastric bypass procedures involve reducing the size of the stomach and bypassing the duodenum (the first part of the small intestine), connecting it to the jejunum further down the gut. This significantly reduces the amount of nutrients (and hence calories) that are absorbed and as a result leads to greater weight loss than procedures that simply reduce the stomach volume.

There have been numerous reports of the effect of such weight-loss procedures on people with diabetes. In one report, 72 per cent of people with diabetes had reversed their diabetes after two years, and half of these were still not diabetic after ten years. There were similar improvements in other aspects of the metabolic syndrome, such as high blood pressure and cholesterol levels.

Research from Italy has described the reversal of diabetes in people who underwent a type of gastric bypass operation. As is common after gut surgery, patients were unable to eat and were fed through a drip for the first six days after their operation (a total of 1,800 calories per day). What was significant was that by day seven they had already lost an average of 6 kg (13 pounds) in weight and their glucose tolerance test was normal. This weight loss and reversal of diabetes could not have been the result of the operation as it mostly occurred before they had started eating, so they were not even using their new gut. It was more likely their diabetes had reversed as they were unable to eat and instead were on a drip which did not give them enough calories to maintain their pre-operation body weight. The weight loss would have been accompanied by loss of fat from the liver (which, as we learnt in Chapter 2, is an important cause of insulin resistance), which in turn would have enabled insulin to work more effectively in reducing the 'leak' of glucose from the liver into the bloodstream, thus reducing their blood glucose levels to reverse their diabetes.

Professor Roy Taylor of Newcastle University set out to examine the effect of sudden weight loss on both the fat in the liver and on blood glucose levels in 11 people with established type 2 diabetes.[14] He did this by performing various blood tests and MRI scans to look at the liver and the pancreas of the people in the study. They were then asked to follow a strict 600 calories per day (liquid) diet for eight weeks. What he found was quite remarkable: within a week blood glucose levels returned to normal and this was accompanied by a big reduction in the amount of fat in the liver. Over the next few weeks, the fat content in the pancreas also reduced. By eight weeks, the people in the project had lost around 15 kg (33 pounds) on average, the pancreas was producing insulin normally and the liver was no longer resistant to the effect of insulin – the leaky tap had a new washer. Taken together, these changes meant that the people in the study no longer had diabetes.

These experiments confirmed the theory that type 2 diabetes is related to the amount of fat in the liver and in the pancreas. What was even more exciting was the discovery that a big reduction in calorie intake could reverse the disease process. This was great news because it meant that if you had recently been diagnosed with type 2 diabetes, then, by reducing your calorie intake and weight, there was a chance that you could become free from diabetes. Initially, I heard a number of doctors dismiss Professor Taylor's work on the basis that he only looked at a small number of people; that they were required to follow a very low-calorie diet, which is not sustainable in the longer term; and that, after the study, some people regained weight and became diabetic again. But this rather misses the point in that this was an experiment that proved that weight loss, without bariatric surgery, could lead to reversal of diabetes. Of course, a very low-calorie diet is not a sustainable long-term way of managing type 2 diabetes as you would eventually waste away. The point was, for the first time, we had evidence that lifestyle change could reverse type 2 diabetes.

At about the same time as this research was being done, I was seeing people with type 2 diabetes in my clinics at the Royal Bournemouth Hospital in the UK. I had become very interested in the new drugs that came on stream in 2007. One in particular was being touted as the latest wonder drug. It was called exenatide (or Byetta) and promised not only to help reduce blood glucose levels in people with diabetes, but also to help them lose weight. Some other diabetes medications, such as insulin or sulfonylureas, may help reduce glucose levels in the short term in people with type 2 diabetes, but they are very often also associated with extra weight gain. So a drug that reduced sugar levels and helped people lose weight really was revolutionary. There was also great anticipation, as the previous 'wonder drug', troglitazone, launched ten years previously, had had to be withdrawn after just a few weeks after a number of people developed severe liver problems within a short time of taking it – and some died.

At that time, while we were all encouraged to ask people to make lifestyle changes to control type 2 diabetes (so called 'diet and exercise'), I had come to accept that lifestyle changes didn't work, as all too often people came back requiring more medication. This was consistent with what we knew from the UK Prospective Diabetes Study, that type 2 diabetes is a condition that just gets worse over time. I guess like most doctors at the time, I had come to see my role as prescribing the best (or least bad) treatment available to help people keep their blood glucose levels under control. And at last, I thought, we had a drug that really would make a difference. The problem was that Byetta had to be given by injection, twice a day, which immediately put many people off. Then, some people found it made them nauseous, which also put them off. But that still left quite a few, who seemed to do really well. They didn't mind injecting themselves twice a day. They might have experienced some nausea, but they saw that as a positive thing as it reduced their appetite. Their glucose levels started coming down, and when I saw them again six months later, many had lost weight. For those who were unwilling to inject, or could not tolerate Byetta, there was another new drug available in tablet form, called sitagliptin (Januvia). This also came with all sorts of promises, but it was acknowledged that it wasn't as effective as Byetta. I prescribed it to people who didn't want to, or couldn't, take Byetta.

Fast-forward another year, and I was seeing patient after patient who had been prescribed sitagliptin, and nothing seemed to have changed. Their diabetes was still out of control and they had not lost any weight. It was for me a very depressing situation. Even more depressing was that many who were injecting themselves with Byetta also seemed to have nothing to show for it a year later, even if they had initially made gains. I was not just depressed, I was profoundly disheartened to the extent that I felt cheated by all the advance publicity that had convinced me this was such a great drug. Out of that negativity came one of the most exciting changes in my practice ever. It was also actually very simple – for the first time in my career (by then I had been a doctor for over 20 years), I actually asked people with type 2 diabetes what they ate. Very simply, in a few short questions. I asked, 'What do you like to eat for breakfast... for lunch... and for your evening meals?' My supplementary questions were, 'And if you get hungry between meals, what do like to have for a snack?' and, 'What do you like to drink?' The answers were a complete revelation.

Firstly, it struck me that so many people were eating variations on the same themes. Nearly everyone had cereal of some description, or toast, or both for breakfast. Sometimes with jam or honey on the toast. Lunch was usually a sandwich, perhaps with a packet of crisps and/or some fruit. Evening meals often included large portions of rice, pasta or potatoes. Many had been told that a banana was a great snack, many also ate biscuits or cakes. Fortunately, very few people added sugar to their tea or coffee, and people mostly used diet fizzy drinks rather than the sugary versions. Otherwise, nearly every meal was based around starchy carbohydrates and many snacks were high in sugar, including fruit. It seems obvious that sugar will push up the blood sugar level, but what people are less aware of is that starch, found in foods such as bread, potatoes, pasta, rice and cereals, is essentially sugar molecules joined together, or 'holding hands' as my colleague Dr David Unwin so nicely puts it. Within seconds of passing one's lips, they begin to let go of each other and become glucose. That meant that almost every time my patients put food in their mouth, that food would push up their blood glucose levels.

In a sense, I should not have been surprised that this is what so many people with type 2 diabetes were eating. After all, the standard advice at the time was to base all meals on starchy carbohydrates, to eat at least five portions of fruit and veg each day and that no food was off limits (including up to 50 g of added sugar per day – that's over 12 teaspoons!), as long as you eat in moderation.

Quite quickly it dawned on me: what chance does any drug have in controlling blood glucose levels in someone who is constantly eating foods that push up those levels? And, given that we now understood that the main problems in type 2 diabetes result from high glucose and high insulin levels, this eating pattern would just aggravate exactly the issues that are the main problem – by keeping glucose levels high, the body will produce more and more insulin to try to reduce them. That will increase the amount of fat in the liver, leading to insulin resistance. Insulin resistance means the glucose levels will remain high, causing the body to try to produce even more insulin… quickly setting up a vicious circle that just makes the problem worse.

As soon as that penny had dropped, I immediately started saying to patients, 'Your blood glucose levels are high and at this stage I would usually suggest that we need to add in another medication. However, if you are willing to make some changes to your diet, we may be able to avoid that.' I gave some examples, such as eggs or plain Greek yoghurt for breakfast, soup or salad at lunch, and to replace starchy foods with leafy green vegetables with their main meals – and try to avoid all sugary foods, including sweet fruits such as banana and pineapple. I didn't use any diet sheets, fancy handouts, dietitians or websites. Just those few words. Now I wish I had provided written resources as it has been known for a long time that many people cannot recall the detail of a consultation with a doctor within minutes of leaving the consultation room. But I did start writing to all my patients, rather than just to their GPs, after each consultation, summarizing the recommendations, so they did get a written record.

I waited to see what happened…

As the months passed, more and more people would come back and say that they had made some of the changes I had suggested.

Some felt unable to continue and so had gone back to their previous way of eating, but others were able to stick with some changes and saw significant reductions in their blood glucose levels. And some went the whole way and were not only able to reduce their glucose levels, but also able to reduce their medications at the same time, including some people who actually came off insulin, having been on it for several years. I was amazed! The only way that I could explain this was that the diet changes they had made had helped to stop the vicious circle that drives type 2 diabetes and had started to reverse that disease process – even if they still had the condition.

Given that we now understood that excess insulin is the main problem in prediabetes and type 2 diabetes, it seemed logical that reducing carbohydrate intake would reduce the blood glucose levels. That, in turn, would mean the body did not need to produce so much insulin, thus reducing the level of insulin in the blood, which could gradually lead to the excess fat in the liver being reduced – thus reversing the diabetes disease process. Could it be, therefore, that reducing carbohydrates would also be able to reverse diabetes?

At that time, I worked in a specialist diabetes centre and most of the patients I saw had type 1 diabetes or longstanding type 2 diabetes, often with complex complications; most people with type 2 diabetes were generally managed by their GP or practice nurse. But now I had seen enough evidence that carbohydrate restriction had really helped some of my own patients with type 2 diabetes. I had also started exploring internet forums such as diabetes.co.uk and and found that many people with diabetes were also finding success using the low-carbohydrate approach. In 2011, I was asked if I would consider writing a book to help people with type 2 diabetes manage their condition. I jumped at the opportunity and said that I would, as long as I could include my ideas about reducing carbohydrates to help reverse it. I wanted to get the message out to as many people as possible. The book did not make any promises but explained the hypothesis and the reasons why reducing carbohydrates might help. That book, *Reverse Your Diabetes: The Step-By-Step Plan to Take Control of Type 2 Diabetes*, was eventually published in 2014. I waited with bated breath to see how it would be received. I didn't have to wait long, as within a few weeks, people were writing reviews to explain how they had put my recommendations into practice and had lost weight and seen their glucose levels improve dramatically. Within a few months, people contacted me to tell me how delighted they were that they had managed to reverse their diabetes... it was the proof I was seeking.

Almost exactly six months after the book was published, in May 2015, I came across a TED Talk given by Dr Sarah Hallberg, a doctor in the US who specializes in the treatment of obesity. Her talk was entitled, 'Reversing type 2 diabetes starts with ignoring the guidelines'.[15] It is well worth watching, as she explains, very eloquently, how carbohydrates in food can actually make things worse in type 2 diabetes, and how reducing them (and thereby going against the guidelines that recommend eating carbohydrates regularly) can reverse it.

Later that year, I was put in touch with Dr David Unwin, who in 2013 had started advising his own patients to adopt a low-carb diet. He is a GP based in Southport, a town in the north-west of England, and he had many patients with type 2 diabetes in his practice who just didn't seem to be doing very well. Then along came a woman whom he barely recognized, even though she had been his patient for many years. She had lost some weight, well, actually a lot of weight. She rather sheepishly told him that she had done so by ignoring his advice and, instead of following a low-fat diet, had started a low carb-diet. He was so impressed by how well she had done that he began to advise his patients with type 2 diabetes to reduce the carbohydrates in their food. His approach was very similar to mine, to point out that all starches are broken down in the body into sugar and therefore push up blood glucose levels. He would help people learn which foods contain sugar and starches and provide advice on alternatives they could eat. And like me, he found that this helped many of his patients lose weight, reduce their medications, and in some cases reverse their diabetes. I was no longer feeling so alone in my approach!

The evidence that type 2 diabetes can be reversed

After the success of Professor Roy Taylor's research showing that rapid weight loss can reverse type 2 diabetes, Diabetes UK funded a large study called DiRECT (DIabetes REmission Clinical Trial) to see if a very low-calorie diet could work as a treatment for people with type 2 diabetes – i.e. to put the research into practice. The study recruited people with type 2 diabetes, aged 65 or under, who were not on insulin and who had had the condition for less than 6 years. These were considered to be the groups most likely to be able to achieve remission of type 2 diabetes. They were asked to follow a very low-calorie diet (800 calories per day) for up to 12 weeks. The diet essentially involved using meal-replacement powders (carefully designed to provide all essential vitamins and minerals) to make up as 'shakes', together with vegetables and plentiful fluids. When they started, all diabetes and blood pressure medications were stopped. Standard meals were gradually reintroduced and people were advised to reduce their portion sizes and avoid refined carbohydrates in the future, to increase the chance of their diabetes staying in remission.

In 2019, the research was published. It showed that, after one year, participants had lost an average of 10 kg (22 pounds) in weight, and their HbA1c had reduced by 10 mmol/mol (0.9 per cent). In total, 46 per cent were in remission from their diabetes. After the second year, there was a slight increase in average weight and HbA1c and the number whose diabetes was in remission had reduced to 36 per cent, which meant that during the second year, diabetes had returned in a quarter of those who had gone into remission.[16] This highlights the importance of people not returning to their previous eating habits, otherwise the diabetes will return. While some people like the idea of a short, sharp shock to induce rapid weight loss, it is not for everyone. I heard a participant in this study speak at a large diabetes conference. They were successful in reversing their diabetes but found the very low-calorie diet extremely difficult, especially when the rest of their family carried on eating normal meals. I know of someone else who followed a similar plan using real food instead of replacements, as described by Dr Michael Mosley in his book *The 8-Week Blood Sugar Diet*. He found that he could not function normally in his job while on the low-calorie diet, and he actually fainted twice, for the first time in his life. So maybe it is not for everyone.

Meanwhile, Dr Sarah Hallberg in the US was working on a different approach. She headed up a team at Virta Health that was testing a very low-carbohydrate, ketogenic diet. In this study, people with type 2 diabetes were asked to restrict their carbohydrates to less than 30 g each day. This essentially means excluding all sugary and starchy foods and getting just a few carbs from non-starchy vegetables and berries. It is therefore quite restrictive. As this is not designed to be a low-calorie diet, it also means increasing the fat content in the diet to make up for the lack of carbs and to encourage the body to switch away from using glucose as its main fuel, and instead to use fat. Burning fat for energy leads to the production of ketones (chemicals produced in the liver when it breaks down fats) and participants in the study were asked to measure the ketone level in their blood as a means of ensuring that their body had switched to fat-burning. This involves using a test strip and meter, very similar to the devices used to measure blood glucose levels. They published their results in 2018. After one year, people in this study had lost an average of 15 kg (33 pounds) in weight and their HbA1c had reduced by 15 mmol/mol (1.3 per cent). In total, 59 per cent achieved remission. In the US, it is customary for people who are on metformin to stay on it even when they are in remission, as it is thought that its effect in making the body's insulin more effective is beneficial for their overall health and helps keep them in remission. Therefore, nearly two-thirds of people in remission were still on metformin. After two years, there was a slight increase in average weight and HbA1c, but 53 per cent were still in remission, meaning that diabetes had reappeared in only 10 per cent.[17] As this diet is designed to be a long-term, permanent change in eating behaviour, these data suggest that for those who are able to live within its restrictions, it can be very effective in helping them achieve remission and stay in remission. As so many people stayed on metformin, we cannot directly compare the results with the low-calorie DiRECT study. However, the fact that only 10 per cent relapsed in the second year would seem to suggest it is a more successful approach in the longer term, than the short, sharp shock low-calorie approach. Some doctors have expressed concern that, as the very low-carbohydrate, ketogenic diet has a high fat content, this could increase cholesterol levels in the blood. While this did happen, the HDL (high-density lipoprotein) cholesterol that is generally considered healthy increased much more than the more harmful LDL (low-density lipoprotein) cholesterol, and triglycerides (another type of harmful fat in the blood) significantly reduced. The overall impact was to make the cholesterol make-up in the blood more, not less, healthy. (See Chapter 16 for more details on the different types of cholesterol.)

I think that a very low-carbohydrate diet can be a very effective way for people to achieve remission of type 2 diabetes, especially if they are significantly overweight, and a number of my patients now use this approach. But it is not the approach that I recommend for everyone at the start, for four main reasons:

1. Everyone is different, and I do not believe that 'one size fits all', that is, not everyone needs to reduce their carbohydrate intake by so much to achieve remission.
2. My underlying philosophy is to offer people information and then to encourage them to set their own goal in respect of their diabetes or prediabetes, and to make their own choice as to what changes they wish to make to achieve that goal.
3. Dietary changes should be seen not as a short-term fix but as a permanent change in eating behaviours. And to achieve that, it is essential that any changes are sustainable – meaning that you can keep them up for the long term.
4. I want to minimize the chance of setbacks, or of people feeling they have failed; a feeling that many people with type 2 diabetes will have experienced, especially about diet. Telling people that they must adopt a big change to their diet in one go may work well for some, but for others who cannot keep up with it, there is the risk of feeling a failure.

Therefore, I encourage people to make changes at their own pace, according to what they feel they can manage. Some people might start with one change – for example, just giving up drinking fruit juice. They may see what a big impact that has on their blood glucose levels and be encouraged to make another change; they may also then be so motivated and encouraged that they decide to cut out other foods. Some might get to the stage where they stop eating something – for example, bread – but they miss it so much that they decide to have one slice a day, in the overall context of a reduced-carb diet. Others will realize that they can manage without it and then cut out all starchy foods to adopt a very low-carbohydrate diet.

Earlier, I explained how Dr David Unwin started to advise a low-carbohydrate diet in 2013. A few years later, I visited him to see how he did it. Within his usual ten-minute consultation, he would introduce the idea, ask people if they were willing to try to give up sugar, and provide information about the sort of changes that would be needed to achieve this and reduce starches. He did not specify a certain amount that people should or should not eat. Later on, he produced what have now become quite famous infographics – postcards that explain the effect of eating certain foods by comparing them with the effect of teaspoons of sugar. These showed, for example, that a slice of white bread could have a similar effect on your blood glucose as eating three teaspoons of sugar.

In 2020, Dr Unwin published data on 128 people with type 2 diabetes who he had followed up on after providing this advice. After nearly two years, they had lost an average of over 8 kg (over 17 pounds) in weight and their HbA1c had reduced by 17.5 mmol/mol (1.6 per cent). They also reduced their blood pressure and cholesterol levels, just by reducing their carbs. Many came off medication and 46 per cent achieved remission of their diabetes. What was also encouraging was that people over the age of 65 did just as well as those who were younger, and those with diabetes for longer than six years also did very well (remember these groups were excluded from the DiRECT trial).[18]

In Chapter 4, I explained that I was invited to set up a programme in Bermuda, where the food and physical environments contribute to a very high rate of type 2 diabetes and obesity. Even in that environment, people were able to reverse their diabetes. We studied 100 people who were followed up for a year, many of whom had very high glucose levels at the start. They lost an average of 3.4 kg (7.5 pounds) in weight and reduced HbA1c by 12 mmol/mol (1.1 per cent). Nearly half reduced their diabetes medication and 12 per cent achieved drug-free remission of their diabetes. Many also reduced their blood pressure medication, some no longer needed tablets for back pain, gout, acid reflux or erectile dysfunction. All great added bonuses, especially as, even for people with health insurance, medications are very expensive in Bermuda.

You may have noticed that, although the average reduction in HbA1c in Bermuda was similar to other studies, the weight loss was less and relatively fewer people achieved full remission. This is partly explained by the fact that many people had a very high HbA1c level when they came into the programme, and so the average was much higher than in the other research studies I have quoted. Despite good reductions in HbA1c, this was not enough to bring many people's blood sugar level below the 48 mmol/mol (6.5 per cent) that is required for remission. Nevertheless, we know that any reduction is beneficial for longer-term health. Bermuda is an ethnically diverse society, with around two-thirds of the population of African heritage and one-third white European. We know that there are metabolic differences between these populations, and these, together with the very high consumption of sugary foods and drinks, could also have influenced the results in some way. Nevertheless, it was very heartening to know that the programme was effective in helping so many people improve their overall health and reduce their need for medication.

In 2019, one of the doctors who I worked with in Bermuda, Dr Daniel Katambo, returned from Bermuda to his native Kenya. Daniel was so keen to provide a service in his home country that he worked as an unpaid volunteer to develop and deliver a low-carbohydrate programme in Nairobi. He did this both in a private clinic as well as at a charity that provides care for people on very low incomes, often living in slums. Although follow-up was curtailed due to the Covid pandemic, he was able to show that the low-carbohydrate approach helped many of his patients achieve remission of type 2 diabetes. Both he and I were really excited to see that the results among the low-income participants were just as good as for those who attended the private clinic. This had huge implications, as the very poor are not able to afford medical care, nor to pay for the medications used to treat diabetes. They also have a traditional diet that is high in carbohydrates yet were still able to make changes that they could afford, that enabled them to get their condition under control, and in many cases reverse their diabetes. This is really encouraging for policymakers, as well as for people with type 2 diabetes, in Kenya and other lower-income countries, many of which are on the cusp of an explosion of type 2 diabetes, as their populations adopt the lifestyles that have caused so much ill health in many Western countries. I have since made links with doctors in the Democratic Republic of the Congo, Malaysia,

North America and Australia, who all report that the low-carb approach works.

The message is, regardless of where you live, your ethnicity, your income level or the extent to which your current diet is based on carbohydrates, if you are willing to make changes to your diet, then it is possible to reduce your blood glucose levels and lose weight, while also reducing your need for medication – not just for diabetes but also for high blood pressure and other conditions. And for some, that will result in achieving remission of type 2 diabetes or prediabetes.

What is the right approach for you?

To summarize, there are a number of dietary approaches that have been shown to reverse the diabetes disease process and help people achieve remission of prediabetes or type 2 diabetes. These are:

- a very-low calorie diet to induce rapid weight loss, followed by a diet low in sugars and refined carbohydrates;
- a low-carbohydrate diet (50–130 g of carbohydrate per day); or
- a very low-carbohydrate, ketogenic diet (less than 50 g of carbs per day).

The definitions of a very low or low-carbohydrate diet are rather arbitrary and I would not get too bogged down by them. At the end of the day, the diet that works best for you is the one that you can stick with, whatever its composition.

In early 2021, I conducted an online survey as I was interested to find out which option people chose and how well they did. Of 79 people who replied, 38 chose the low-carbohydrate option, 33 the very low-carbohydrate, ketogenic diet, and 8 the very low-calorie approach.

The 38 who chose the low-carbohydrate approach lost an average of 16.9 kg (37 pounds) in weight. Of the total, 11 subsequently reduced their carbohydrate intake to below 50 g per day, and 9 of these achieved drug-free remission of their diabetes. Of the 27 who stayed on up to 130 g of carbs per day, 13 achieved drug-free remission and 12 did not. However, this group still lost a lot of weight, and many were able to reduce their medications.

The 33 who chose the very low-carbohydrate, ketogenic diet at the outset lost an average of 17.3 kg (38 pounds) in weight. In total, 25 achieved drug-free remission of their diabetes, including 2 who had increased their carb intake to above 50 g per day.

The 8 who chose the very low-calorie approach lost an average of 15.1 kg (33 pounds) in weight and 6 achieved drug-free remission of their diabetes, having adopted a low-carbohydrate or very low-carbohydrate diet within a few months. The results are shown in Figure 3.

Figure 3: Remission of type 2 diabetes on different diets

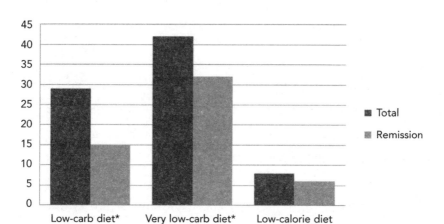

* Refers to final chosen diet option.

Now it is important to remember that this information was submitted by people via an online survey, and I have no way of checking how accurate it is. Nevertheless, it provides a useful snapshot of the approaches that people took, and of how they did. It suggests that all three approaches are effective in helping people lose weight and achieve remission of diabetes. The low-carbohydrate approach was slightly less effective at achieving remission than the very low-carbohydrate or very low-calorie approaches, but still enabled over 50 per cent to achieve remission of their diabetes. Many others, while not achieving remission, were able to lose weight and come off some of their medications.

A similar survey of people with prediabetes was completed by 18 people: 6 out of the 8 on a low-carbohydrate diet, and 9 out of the 10 on a very low-carbohydrate diet, achieved remission of their prediabetes. Although the number of responses was much smaller, this snapshot suggests that both approaches are successful at reversing prediabetes.

The very low-calorie diet is suitable for people who want to lose a lot of weight in a short period of time. However, while you are on the low-calorie regime, it does mean abstaining from normal meals and/or eating very low-calorie meals that are likely to be different from what others in your household eat. It is also essential that if you choose this option, you do not return to your previous diet once normal eating resumes. It is recommended to reduce refined carbohydrates. This option can therefore be regarded as a long-term low-carbohydrate diet, preceded by a very low-calorie phase to kick-start weight loss.

The low-carbohydrate approach can be achieved by removing as much sugar as possible from your diet, while still enjoying small portions of starchy foods. It is less restrictive than the other options and, by allowing each person to make their own decisions about which foods to reduce, is potentially more sustainable. As we saw from my online survey, some people then choose to reduce to a very low-carbohydrate diet.

The very low-carbohydrate (ketogenic) diet requires reducing carbohydrate intake to less than 50 g per day. This means removing all sugars and starches and may be too restrictive for some people, or too big a change to make in one go. If you choose to adopt a very low-carbohydrate diet, it will be important to review your medications with your doctor or nurse to ensure that neither your blood glucose levels nor your blood pressure fall too low.

There are other dietary approaches that claim to reverse type 2 diabetes, including a low-fat vegan diet. This is necessarily higher in carbohydrates than the other approaches, but sugar and refined carbohydrates are still discouraged, and carbohydrate intake is advised to be mainly wholegrains. I am sure this can work for some people, particularly if it helps them lose a lot of weight. Indeed, any approach that enables a person to lose weight, and keep it off, can potentially lead to reversal of prediabetes or type 2 diabetes. However, I am not aware of any research studies that have confirmed the low-fat vegan diet is as effective as the other approaches I have mentioned.

It is for you to decide which approach is right for you. If you are not sure, then I would recommend starting by trying to reduce your sugar intake as much as you can, and then to reduce your intake of starches. In Chapter 6, I will explain how to go about achieving that.

ALISON'S STORY

I work as an accountant in the south of England. I was diagnosed with prediabetes at the age of 36 and I have been following a low-carb diet for the two years since. After about five months the prediabetes had reversed, and it is still 'in remission'. I've no idea how long I was prediabetic, but it could have been a few years, I think.

Before I was diagnosed, I felt I was in good health. I did a lot of exercise, mainly running and cycling, and was generally happy other than occasional work stress. I probably wasn't the fittest I'd ever been but I considered myself in good shape. I felt I had to work hard not to become overweight and, on several occasions, I would go on a diet, losing several kilos (5 or 6 pounds), then gradually putting weight back on (repeated over and over). I only got the diagnosis because I was concerned about irregular periods.

When I was diagnosed, my HbA1c was 44 (6.2 per cent) and I weighed 56 kg (123 pounds). I was given general advice to lose weight and exercise more which I didn't think seemed relevant (as I did that already). I looked at much more overweight people and thought 'why me?' I received a letter from my GP practice with an invite to a diet class but I decided not to go. My BMI was probably near the top of normal but not overweight. I also felt I had been getting healthy eating advice all my life and that hadn't prevented me from being prediabetic.

I was aware of the low-carb diet as I heard about it from my dad. He had been diagnosed prediabetic at the age of 74 and about a year before me and had been recommended the *Reverse Your Diabetes Diet* book by a friend. He went on to successfully reverse his prediabetes. I was previously very sceptical about people saying carbs were unhealthy, as a lot of runners and cyclists actively carb load, but I was willing to give it a try as I didn't feel I had help from anywhere else. Also, I saw online so many people saying it had worked for them!

I tend to be a bit all or nothing, so I changed a lot in one go. Sweets, chocolate, cakes, biscuits weren't a big part of my diet anyway but were banned henceforth. I had a menu plan and tried some of the meals on there. Generally, I replaced the rice/pasta/potato with vegetables like broccoli or cauliflower. I swapped the breakfast porridge for eggs and bacon or avocado, and swapped the lunch sandwich for soup or salad and cheese or fish. I used the 'MyFitnessPal' app to count the carbs and try to stay around the 100 g per day mark. The app automatically adjusts when you do exercise, so it was a bit of an experiment to manage hunger and carb intake while trying to continue with my running. I stopped drinking beer as it has a lot of carbs so either had sparkling water or a dry white wine instead. I lost 3 kg (7 pounds) in weight and my HbA1c came down to 33 (5.2 per cent).

I found the low-carb diet easier than I expected. I have been on diets for years (restricting calories and eating a 'balanced' diet) and have felt hungry all the time and this was definitely better. I lost weight quickly and that gave me motivation. I used to really enjoy baking cakes and I had to give this up as it's too much temptation (even if I've been on a long run or bike ride). I don't miss it now, but it was hard at first. I guess looking back the hardest bit was actually getting enough to eat, which sounds odd, but I had to take out a lot of the calorie-rich foods and needed to work out how to replace them. I wanted to keep up with my running and not make myself ill.

I missed home-made bread and cakes but I don't think I craved them. Sometimes if I really craved something I would just eat it and not feel bad about it. I noticed how hungry I would feel a few hours after and it reminded me of what life used to be like, so it was a motivation to keep these 'treat' foods as rare occurrences. I realized they are not really 'treats' because they are a way to ruin your health, but I am pragmatic about it and accept that sometimes it is going to happen as I am not perfect! I tried to focus on foods that I could eat. I have one or two squares of 85 per cent dark chocolate at the end of the day – and that is my treat.

My husband is really supportive, and while not all my family understand it, they don't question it – so it's not a problem if I ask for different food at a social gathering. I warn people in advance to try to reduce the awkwardness.

I didn't really talk to my doctor about the low-carb diet because they just told me to go on the course they had recommended if I was worried about the diagnosis. The doctor gave the impression it was nothing to worry about; he said, 'it just means you're at a higher risk of developing diabetes in the future', like there was nothing to be done!

I feel like my health is the same, but I feel glad I have taken some control of it. I now have freedom from the dieting/weight-gain cycle and peace of mind that I hope I will not get diabetes in the future.

———————————————

CHAPTER 6

There is such a thing as a 'diabetic diet'

Myth: There is no such thing as a diabetic diet – just eat healthily. **Fact:** Making dietary changes is the natural way to reverse prediabetes and type 2 diabetes.

The curse of 'healthy eating'

In Chapter 5, we discussed the different dietary approaches that have been shown to help reverse prediabetes and type 2 diabetes. By definition, therefore, these are diets that will specifically help anyone with these conditions. In old-fashioned terminology, they would each be called a 'diabetic diet'.

One of the biggest myths in the past 30 years or so is that there is no such thing as a 'diabetic diet'. Go back to the 1980s and everyone who had diabetes, along with most doctors and nurses, understood what a diabetic diet was. They might not have known the precise details, but essentially they would know it was a diet very low in sugar, and where starches are strictly controlled – essentially a low-carbohydrate diet.

Throughout history, until almost exactly 100 years ago, restricting carbohydrates was the only treatment available for a person with diabetes. With the discovery of insulin in the 1920s, there was for the first time a treatment that could reduce blood glucose levels and enable the body to make use of carbohydrates in the diet. However, even with insulin, it was still recommended to limit carbohydrates, as a person with diabetes cannot handle carbohydrates properly; it is a form of carbohydrate intolerance. In almost any other type of food intolerance, the advice would be to restrict or eliminate those foods which you cannot tolerate. And this was the basis of the standard 'diabetic diet' right up to the 1980s. A few years ago, I met a woman who worked as a nurse with Dr R.D. Lawrence and who lent me her treasured copy of the final edition of his book *The Diabetic ABC: A Practical Book for Patients and Nurses*, published in 1964. Dr Lawrence had type 1 diabetes and was, in 1923, one of the first people in the UK to receive insulin. He then went on to become a specialist in diabetes and in his book describes his recommended diet for people with diabetes.

The basic recommendation for people not on insulin (i.e. most people with type 2 diabetes) was to restrict carbohydrates to about 100 g per day. For people on insulin, it was necessary to have snacks between meals to avoid dangerously low blood glucose levels, as the insulins available then were rather primitive compared with today, and there was no way to measure your blood glucose level. That increased the total carbohydrates to 150 g each day. He followed such a diet and lived to the age of 76 after a long and illustrious career and 45 years of living with diabetes, which was quite remarkable for those days.

Yet, by the time I trained in diabetes in the early 1990s, the message was 'there is no such thing as a diabetic diet'. As a result, there were no longer diet sheets to advise people on what to eat (although people kept asking for one). After all, we were told, people with diabetes just need to eat a healthy diet. That meant they needed to follow the healthy eating rules that apply to the whole population. By then, that meant a high-fibre, low-fat diet, with all meals based on starchy carbohydrates.

The reason why national guidelines had changed was because rising rates of heart disease were thought to be related to high cholesterol levels. And high cholesterol levels were thought to be due to fat in the diet: fat was out, and carbs were in. It's (almost) as simple as that. Now even if a high-carb, low-fat diet is a good thing for people with perfect metabolic health (and I think the evidence suggests that it isn't), surely it isn't a good idea for someone with diabetes, whose body by definition cannot tolerate carbohydrates? So why was the advice for people with diabetes changed?

That is a question that I have been asking for some time. During the 2021 lockdown, I gave an online talk about management of type 1 diabetes, in which I suggested that carbohydrate restriction could help people achieve more stable blood glucose levels. (Unlike type 2 diabetes, type 1 diabetes cannot be reversed, and people need to inject insulin; the more carbohydrate you eat, the more insulin you need – so reducing carbohydrate seemed to make sense.) I was asked, 'What is the evidence that a low-carbohydrate diet is effective?' I pointed out that the standard diet advice for people with diabetes, for centuries, was a low-carbohydrate diet. I then asked, 'What was the evidence to suggest a high-carbohydrate diet would be better?' and I did not get a reply. Now you might think that a major change in public health policy, such as the diet advising people with diabetes, would only come about if there was concrete evidence from research projects in large numbers of people to suggest it was the right thing to do. I have yet to find that evidence.

I did find a one-year study that was published in the *Journal of Nutrition* in 1978.[19] It compared two groups of people newly diagnosed with diabetes (presumably type 2 diabetes, although this was not specified) and presumably not on any medication (this, again, was not specified). One group of 54 people were asked to follow a 'low-carbohydrate diet' (of around 150 g of carbohydrate per day) and the other group of 39 people followed a higher-carbohydrate, low-fat diet (around 200 g of carbohydrate per day). The currently recognized definition of a low-carbohydrate diet is less than 130 g of carbohydrate per day, so neither group was really low carb! There were significant differences in the average weight between the groups, and one group had many more men than the other. That means the groups were not 'well matched' and any differences in the results could be because the groups of participants were so different in the first place.

So what did it show? After one year, both groups had lost some weight and reduced their fasting blood glucose levels – with no difference between the groups. The group on the lower-fat diet had a slightly lower total cholesterol level than the lower-carbohydrate group, but then the lower-fat group had started off with lower cholesterol in the first place! Triglyceride levels (which are thought to contribute to heart disease) were very similar in both the groups and we do not know about the levels of HDL (high-density lipoprotein) and LDL (low-density lipoprotein) cholesterol as these were not measured.

In fact, this study tells us very little. It compared two different groups of people, neither of which followed a properly low-carbohydrate diet. There was no difference in weight loss or glucose levels between the groups. Yet it was claimed this meant a high-carbohydrate diet was beneficial for people with diabetes.

The following year, the same researchers published a study on only 14 people with type 2 diabetes.[20] They were asked to follow a high-carbohydrate diet (around 350 g per day) for six weeks. Importantly, sugars were excluded from this diet. They then switched to a lower-carbohydrate diet (around 220 g per day) for six weeks, although by today's definition this would also be classed a high-carbohydrate diet. A sample diet plan was provided that compared the two diets. The main difference seemed to be that the higher-carbohydrate diet included a lot of wholemeal bread, Flora margarine and skimmed milk. The lower-carbohydrate diet included butter, whole milk and egg but less bread (and they had white bread). It also included tinned fruit and ice cream, both of which are high in sugar, and which strangely were not allowed in the higher-carbohydrate diet. Not surprisingly, glucose levels were marginally higher on the 'lower-carbohydrate diet'. Cholesterol levels were also slightly higher on the lower-carbohydrate diet. The report concluded that it was not justifiable to prescribe low-carbohydrate diets for people with diabetes. By the way, it was funded by the Flora Information Service and the International Sugar Research Foundation Inc.

By today's standards, this would not be good enough evidence to change dietary recommendations, but, at the time, when fat was deemed to be bad, it supported the prevailing belief among doctors and policymakers that a high-carbohydrate diet was good, not just for the general population, but also for people with diabetes. This belief appears to have been driven by slight reductions in cholesterol levels, rather than any meaningful benefit in reducing weight or blood glucose levels. And the rest is history. As a result, up until 2011, people with diabetes were advised to base all their meals on starchy carbohydrates. As we learnt in Chapter 2, all starches are converted in the body into glucose, so this means every meal would add glucose into the bloodstream. To make matters worse, the official guidance in the UK also said it was okay for a person with diabetes to include up to 50 g of added sugars in their foods each day (that's over 12 teaspoons!). Wow!

Let's consider what following a recommended 'healthy' diet would do to a person with prediabetes or type 2 diabetes. In the UK, healthy eating is summarized by what is called the 'Eatwell Guide' (see Figure 4) and similar versions exist in other countries, with essentially the same message.

Figure 4: The Eatwell Guide

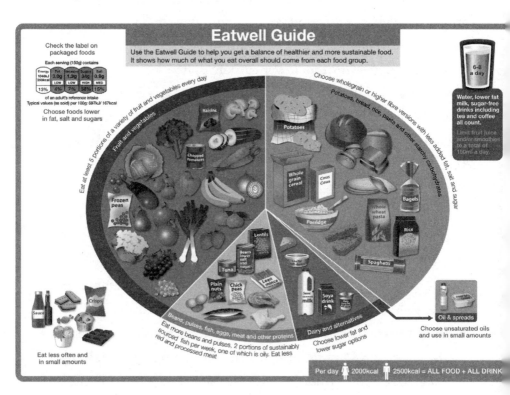

Source: https://www.nhs.uk/live-well/eat-well/the-eatwell-guide (accessed 1 September 2021).

The recommendations can be summarized as follows:

- Eat at least five portions of a variety of fruit and vegetables every day.
- Base meals on potatoes, bread, rice, pasta or other starchy carbohydrates, choosing wholegrain versions where possible.
- Have some dairy or dairy alternatives (such as soy drinks), choosing lower-fat and lower-sugar options.
- Eat some beans, pulses, fish, eggs, meat and other proteins (including two portions of fish every week, one of which should be oily).
- Choose unsaturated oils and spreads and eat in small amounts.
- Drink 6–8 cups/glasses of fluid a day.
- If consuming foods and drinks high in fat, salt or sugar, have these less often and in small amounts.

So, how suitable are these recommendations for a person with diabetes? On the face of it, eating at least five portions of fruit and vegetables seems a good idea – they are healthy, natural and unprocessed foods, aren't they?

For leafy and salad vegetables, the answer is yes – cabbage, courgette (zucchini), cucumber, tomatoes and cauliflower, for example, are all around 3 per cent or less carbohydrate (excluding fibre which strictly speaking is a carbohydrate but is not digested so is not counted). Lettuce, spinach, asparagus, olives and avocado contain even less.

Some root vegetables, such as celeriac or carrots, are pretty low at 7 per cent, whereas potatoes are about 15 per cent. But what about fruit? Bananas can be as much as 20 per cent carbs and grapes are 16 per cent. And raisins are about 75 per cent carbohydrate!

Yet, if you look at the Eatwell Guide, these are all lumped together – in one section. Why? Because this guide was not designed with consideration of its impact on blood glucose levels in mind. According to the Eatwell Guide, these fruit and vegetables are all healthy because they contain fibre and plenty of vitamins and minerals. But a tomato or a few chunks of cucumber will have negligible effect on blood glucose levels, whereas a banana could have a massive impact. A large banana could contain up to 40 g of carbohydrate, and yet many people with diabetes have been recommended this as a healthy snack.

Turning to starches, remember these are just sugar molecules joined together. As soon as they enter your mouth they begin to break down into glucose. So every one of these foods will increase blood glucose levels. Some, such as bread and white rice, will cause a very rapid rise; others, such as pasta, a slower one. Even porridge, which is almost universally believed to be a good thing, contains over 60 per cent carbohydrate and will cause a big and sustained rise in blood glucose. The usual advice is to choose wholegrain versions wherever possible. This is because wholegrains contain more fibre, and this slows down the rise in blood glucose. Yet, in reality, wholegrain versions – whether of bread, rice, pasta or cereal – contain so much carbohydrate that they still have a big impact.

These two sections cover three-quarters of the plate and anyone following the Eatwell Guide will therefore have a high intake of starches and, depending on the fruits chosen, also of sugars. What would this type of diet do to the vicious cycle that is the diabetes disease process? Remember how, in Chapter 2, we learnt that glucose in the bloodstream leads the body to produce insulin. High levels of glucose lead to high levels of insulin. High levels of insulin lead to excess energy being stored as fat in the liver. Fat in the liver leads to glucose leaking out from the liver into the bloodstream, eventually causing type 2 diabetes and – unless something is done to stop it – promoting a continuously revolving vicious cycle. With this understanding that we now have of type 2 diabetes, we can see that the advice to base all meals on starchy carbohydrates just continues that cycle, adding fuel to the flames.

I firmly believe, therefore, that the Eatwell Guide is positively harmful for anyone with diabetes or prediabetes. Given that so many of the population are overweight and obese, and many of those are likely to be developing insulin resistance and heading towards prediabetes, I have also come to the conclusion that a high-carbohydrate, low-fat diet as recommended by the Eatwell Guide is bad advice for the general population. Worse still, it is likely to have contributed to the high rates of obesity, insulin resistance and type 2 diabetes that we are now experiencing.

Thankfully, things have begun to change. The recommendations for people with diabetes in the UK, the US and many other countries no longer recommend that carbohydrates form a certain proportion of meals. Unfortunately, many professionals who treat people with diabetes were trained in the 'high-carbohydrate' era and they often continue to advise, as one example, starchy carbohydrate with every meal. In 2021, the UK government's Scientific Advisory Committee on Nutrition published a report on lower-carbohydrate diets for adults with type 2 diabetes.[21] Within its 347 pages, there are a lot of caveats about gaps in the evidence, so that they could not be certain about some aspects. However, they reported that there was evidence that a lower-carbohydrate diet was better for reducing blood glucose levels and enabling people to come off medication. In fact, in none of the areas looked at did they find that a higher-carbohydrate diet was superior. Diabetes UK does now acknowledge that low-carbohydrate diets can be effective for people with type 2 diabetes, but when discussing reversal of diabetes, the focus is very much on the low-calorie approach (perhaps because Diabetes UK funded the DiRECT study into the low-calorie approach – see Chapter 5). In the US and Canada, the national diabetes associations have come out much more strongly to support low-carbohydrate or very low-carbohydrate diets. By contrast, some authorities – such as in Australia – still refuse to acknowledge that type 2 diabetes can be reversed.

The better choice

I don't think it is any coincidence that rates of obesity and type 2 diabetes have skyrocketed since the 1980s when dietary guidelines recommended a low-fat, high-carbohydrate diet. It makes sense, as the carbohydrates drive the vicious cycle that leads to excess fat in the liver, insulin resistance, prediabetes and then type 2 diabetes.

If you are unlucky enough to be stuck in that cycle, what do you think will help reverse track? It doesn't take a genius to work out that eating foods that do not increase your blood glucose levels would be a good place to start. Now all foods have some effect on blood glucose, but by far the biggest culprits are sugars and starches. Therefore, my first recommendation is to focus on reducing these. As we aren't always aware of what is in processed foods, my second recommendation is to make sure you know what you are eating, and that means as far as possible eating fresh, unprocessed foods. So, what does that mean in practice?

Cutting out sugars

This really is essential, and if you were one of my patients, one of my first questions would be to ask you whether you were willing to try to cut out sugars as much as possible. Minimizing sugars has to be part of a low-carbohydrate or very low-carbohydrate diet.

Remember that, by definition, diabetes is a condition of intolerance to glucose. If you have coeliac disease or gluten intolerance you are advised, instructed even, not to eat any foods that contain gluten. That means consume nothing made with wheat flour, and a whole host of other things – including beer. People are advised to go to great lengths to avoid sharing cutlery or utensils that might have been contaminated with gluten. Uncontrolled coeliac disease can have immediate effects, such as unpleasant gut symptoms, and long-term health consequences – just like diabetes. Similarly, if you have lactose intolerance, you are advised to avoid all dairy products that contain lactose (milk sugar).

Likewise, if you have a peanut allergy, you must avoid all peanuts at all times, otherwise you risk a massive allergic reaction and possible death. Extraordinary measures are sometimes required, such as banning the consumption of peanuts on an aeroplane if someone on board is allergic to them. Diabetes is not like an acute allergy and so that won't happen if you eat sugar. Yet eating sugar on a regular basis will increase your blood glucose level and over time will increase your risk of complications, and that in turn carries an increased risk of death.

Think about it: if you have prediabetes or type 2 diabetes, I would be doing you a considerable disservice in saying that it's okay to eat sugar. Your body just cannot handle it properly.

Does that mean you should never eat sugar? There are some natural sugars in many foods, such as vegetables, dairy products and even eggs, so you cannot avoid it completely. However, as a rule, I recommend trying to eliminate all foods that have added sugars. Apart from the obvious things, such as sugary drinks, sweets, desserts, cakes and biscuits, it will also include many processed foods such as the ubiquitous baked beans. It will also mean avoiding natural sugars or syrups, such as honey, and fruits that are high in sugar, such as bananas, grapes (unless you can limit to just a few), pineapple and large apples, pears and oranges. You may allow yourself to have a small piece of cake to celebrate a special birthday, as a very occasional treat. It will cause your glucose levels to rise, but you are deliberately accepting the risk to share in the moment of celebration.

If you have been led to believe you can eat anything in moderation, and especially if you have been encouraged to eat a lot of fruit as it is healthy, this could entail quite big changes to your current eating pattern.

Reducing starches

Many people say to me that they eat a really good diet and don't have any sugar. But they have large portions of bread, potatoes, rice and pasta. Again, as we read earlier, this was previously the basis of the recommended diet, so you would not be to blame for doing so. However, I would now encourage you to think of all these 'white' or 'beige' foods as what they are to your body – lots of sugar molecules holding hands. Some of them, such as white rice, can actually push up your blood glucose level quicker than a bowlful of table sugar. So, it's not that far-fetched to think of a bowl of rice, pasta, breakfast cereal or potatoes as a bowl of sugar. As far as your body is concerned, that is – to all intents and purposes – precisely what it is.

Starch in our diet comes from grains (such as rice, wheat, barley and oats, and anything made from their flour, such as bread or pasta), pulses (including peas, beans and lentils) and root vegetables (including potatoes, parsnip and carrots).

Whether you eat these foods will determine if you follow a low-carbohydrate or very low-carbohydrate diet. A very low-carb diet of less than 50 g per day means excluding starches as well as sugars. Many of us have been brought up to include starch as an integral part of our meals, but that doesn't mean it has to be. It's actually more important that we include protein and fat, as our bodies need these in our diet. We don't actually need to eat any carbohydrate. Of course, our body needs glucose as fuel, but it can make this from other types of nutrients. So have a think about what you could eat instead. Eggs or plain Greek yoghurt for breakfast? Soup or salad for lunch? And for main meals, replace beige with green. Instead of that portion of potato, rice or pasta, fill your plate up with leafy green or salad vegetables instead. If you're following a low-carbohydrate diet of up to 130 g per day, it is still possible to include a small amount of carbs each day – a slice or two of bread, a few new potatoes or a spoonful of pasta or rice.

Healthy fats and protein

If you just reduce carbohydrates but make no other changes to what you eat, you may find that you go hungry. This would be counterproductive as your body would send out signals to drive you to eat and you could then end up eating whatever is to hand, which could well be something containing carbohydrate. So, if you are reducing carbohydrates, make sure you fill up enough with other types of foods.

This is where protein and healthy fats come in. I generally suggest increasing the portion of protein in your meals. Protein is found in meat, fish, eggs, cheese, pulses and nuts. Adding healthy fats can also make meals more filling. As we will explore in Chapter 7, fat is no longer the baddie that we once believed, responsible for heart attacks and many other ailments. Naturally occurring fats – for example, in dairy products – are now considered healthy again, as are oily fish, nuts, avocados and olives. Adding some of these can make a salad into a really filling meal. Fat has virtually no effect on blood glucose or insulin levels. Protein has some effect, but much less than carbohydrates. Therefore, after eating a meal of fat and protein, there is no surge in insulin to make you hungry again a short time later. In fact, quite the opposite. Meals that contain fat and protein stay in the stomach for longer so that you feel fuller for longer after eating them. If you do get peckish, try having a hard-boiled egg or a sardine from a tin. Both inexpensive, nutritious, real foods. And both guaranteed to kill your hunger. So much so that it will be almost impossible to eat a second one. Now you can't say that about biscuits.

What about calories?

Traditional diets that aim to help people lose weight are based on the principle that, if you take in fewer calories in food and drink than you use up with physical activity, then you will lose weight. This is the basis for all low-calorie diets. Each gram of fat contains 9 calories, whereas each gram of protein or carbohydrate contains 4 calories. Therefore, the logic goes, we should eat less fat and more carbohydrates, hence the idea of a low-fat, high-carb diet. But this misses an important point. It's actually quite difficult to eat a large amount of high fat foods, such as butter or cream, as they fill you up very quickly – whereas it is very easy to eat a large bowl of pasta, so you may end up eating more calories in a high-carb meal.

There is, I believe, another flaw in the argument for a low-fat, high-carb diet. And that is the role of insulin. I would imagine that three tablespoons of double (heavy) cream is, by anyone's standards, a very big portion. That contains just over 200 calories from fat and less than a gram (4 calories) of sugar and will have very little effect on the level of glucose in the blood or the insulin produced in the pancreas. However, just a moderate portion of 150 g of rice also contains about 200 calories (from 50 g of carbohydrate). That amount of carbohydrate will potentially increase the glucose in the blood by as much as 15 mmol/l (270 mg/dl), and so the pancreas will release a large amount of insulin to avoid that happening. Insulin is the fat storage hormone, and so as well as thinking about the impact of calories eaten, we also need to consider what effect those calories have on the level of insulin in the blood. Therefore, 200 calories from a small portion of rice will have a much bigger impact on your insulin levels, and your fat stores, than a whopping three tablespoons of double (heavy) cream. A further flaw is that some foods actually require more energy to digest them than others. Protein requires up to 30 per cent of its calories to digest it, whereas carbohydrate requires about 10 per cent. So, if you eat 200 calories as protein (as in a 200 g (7 oz) steak, for example), 60 of those calories are burned off in the digestion process, meaning your body only gets to use 140 of them. Whereas only 20 calories are burned off digesting the carbs in our small portion of rice. These flaws in the low-calorie argument have led many of us to believe that a calorie in rice or sugar is much more harmful than a calorie in steak or cream, or – put another way – 'a calorie is not a calorie'.

It is undoubtedly the case that if you significantly reduce your calorie intake, say to 800 calories a day, then you will lose weight. But many people find that they can also lose a lot of weight just by reducing the carbohydrate in their diet. Replacing starchy carbs with green vegetables will reduce insulin levels, which is key to losing weight by reversing the vicious cycle of the diabetes disease process.

I, therefore, do not suggest that you focus on counting calories. Reducing the carbs will likely reduce them. In a low-carbohydrate diet, it is important to be aware of the low-carb foods that are high in calories, such as cheese or nuts, and to limit your intake if you want to lose weight – but that is probably enough.

If you choose the very low-calorie diet plan in order to reverse your diabetes, then you will need to focus much more on limiting calories. This is not within the scope of this book, but *The 8-Week Blood Sugar Diet* by Dr Michael Mosley and *Carbs & Cals: Very Low Calorie* books provide full details on how to limit to 800 calories a day using real foods, rather than supplements and shakes, as used in the DiRECT study mentioned in Chapter 5. Remember that the very low-calorie diet is for a limited time, typically 8 to 12 weeks, in order to promote rapid weight loss and remission of diabetes. Once you have achieved your desired weight loss, you will likely need to go on to a lower-carbohydrate diet for the long term to stay in remission.

Avoiding processed foods

Many processed foods contain high levels of sugars, harmful trans fats and all sorts of other chemicals that are not real food at all. A good tip for avoiding processed foods is to buy foods that either do not have an ingredients list (such as fresh meat or vegetables) or that have no more than five ingredients.

Using butter or sunflower spread as an example: there is one ingredient in butter (milk), whereas a sunflower spread has 12 ingredients – vegetable oils (45 per cent, made up of sunflower oil (26 per cent), palm oil, linseed oil), water, salt (1 per cent), emulsifiers (mono- and diglycerides of fatty acids, sunflower lecithin), stabilizer (sodium alginate), preservative (potassium sorbate), acidity regulator (lactic acid), vitamin E, flavouring and colour (beta-carotene). Now for many years we have been told that butter is bad for us as it contains saturated fat. The good news is that dairy fat has been shown to be healthy, and the alternative seed oils are not looking so healthy after all! Other types of processed foods include ready meals (especially the cheaper versions) and almost all foods from fast-food restaurants.

In Chapter 11, we will look in more detail at the dietary changes that are most suitable for a person with prediabetes or type 2 diabetes, or – in old-fashioned terms – a diabetic diet. Meanwhile, remember the key messages: cut out sugar, replace beige with green, and eat real foods!

We have two stories to round off this chapter. The first is from Frances who had prediabetes. That's followed by Stewart's account of how he changed his diet to reverse type 2 diabetes.

FRANCES'S STORY

I am 72 years old and was a teacher but had to retire early due to ME (chronic fatigue syndrome) when I was 50. This stayed with me for 7 years and led me to gain over 25 kg (55 pounds) which I could not shift.

I was unable to exercise but I followed what I thought was a healthy low-calorie diet.

I was diagnosed with prediabetes in 2019, when I weighed 89 kg (196 pounds) and my HbA1c was 43 (6.1 per cent). I was offered a free course at Weight Watchers, which I accepted. At this time, my son, daughter-in-law and my husband all followed a low-carbohydrate diet and recommended I try it. I decided to do so, but I also attended WW because I thought the weekly weigh-ins were a good incentive. Although I did not follow the WW diet, the weight loss measured every week made me determined to stick with my low-carbohydrate diet. After six months, I had lost over 13 kg (29 pounds) and my HbA1c had dropped to 39 (5.7 per cent). I decided to continue with a low-carbohydrate diet and after another year I weighed 70 kg (154 pounds), a total weight loss of 19 kg (42 pounds). I have maintained this weight loss for two years and my HbA1c is now 37 (5.5 per cent). My family were very supportive and because I never felt hungry and kept no carbohydrates in the house, I found it relatively easy.

My daughter then started losing weight with a low-carb diet and this was further encouragement for me not to return to my old ways of eating. Having lost and maintained this weight has boosted my confidence. I started walking every day but my energy levels are not as good as I would like them to be, which is perhaps a throwback to my ME.

STEWART'S STORY

My story starts in June 2012 when I was 59 years old. I saw my GP because I had developed a problem with my leg. A blood test showed that I had developed type 2 diabetes. After I was prescribed metformin and simvastatin, I was put in touch with a nurse who advised me to attend a two-day course during which we were given advice on diet and exercise.

Due to my leg problem, exercise was not really a viable option and I was advised to eat a balanced diet of carbohydrates and protein and to cut out fat and of course sugars. I was advised to eat plenty of fruit and vegetables.

I followed this advice for six years during which time my weight increased and my blood glucose level climbed steadily upwards. I was informed that diabetes was a progressive disease and increasing glucose levels was to be expected but this could be countered by increasing medications. As a result, I was eventually taking metformin, sitagliptin, empagliflozin and gliclazide – and yet still my weight and glucose levels increased. I was then advised that insulin would be the next step in my treatment.

In 2020, a new nurse at the practice mentioned that they were looking for volunteers to join a trial to put diabetes into remission by making lifestyle changes. I thought why not. I was fed up with the amount of medication I was taking and had nothing to lose. The trial started in March 2020 at which point my HbA1c level was 63 (7.9 per cent) and my weight was 95 kg (209 pounds). I followed a low-carb diet and after four months my HbA1c was down to 32 (5.1 per cent) and my weight was down to 82 kg (181 pounds). I was able to reduce my medication and needless to say I was delighted. My HbA1c then increased a little to 38 (5.7 per cent), but I was able to stop all my medication apart from metformin. By June 2021, my HbA1c had stabilized at 38 (5.7 per cent) and my weight was 76 kg (167 pounds), a reduction of 19 kg (42 pounds).

With the weight loss I was able to get out and start walking again. I can now go for walks for up to three hours every day and I'm loving it. I have noticed my concentration is much better. Reading books has become a joy again and I feel sure that my brain function has improved.

My biggest hope is that anyone reading this will eventually have a similar story to tell. I wish you all the very best of luck.

CHAPTER 7

You can eat cheese

Myth: Cheese is full of saturated fat and you shouldn't eat it.
Fact: Saturated fat isn't all bad. Better to eat cheese than a biscuit.

Fat has a bad name – literally. As a noun it describes a nutrient in our food, but the same word, as a (pejorative) adjective, describes someone who is overweight. And so it is easy to link the two and think that fat in food causes fat people. Considering what we have learnt about type 2 diabetes arising because of excess fat in the liver, it is easy to think that fat in our food is a bad thing. That could not be further from the truth. Yes, excess liver fat is bad, but that only occurs if we consume too much energy, particularly in the form of carbohydrates. In past centuries, our ancestors would have been really pleased that their body had the ability to store excess energy, as it helped them survive lean times – over winter, for example, when less food was available.

But fat is far more important than just as an energy store. Unlike carbohydrates, we all need fat in our diet. Fat is essential to our survival. It protects most of our internal organs and it enables us to store and use essential vitamins, such as vitamin D. It is therefore necessary to have some fat in our diet. It is true that fat has 8 calories per gram whereas carbohydrate and protein have only 4 calories. However, this does not necessarily mean eating fat means eating more calories. It does, of course, depend on how much fat-containing food you eat. Most high-fat foods (such as butter, cheese or cream) are eaten in quite small portions and consequently will mean less calories on the plate or in a serving than a standard portion of carbohydrates. Even meat that we tend to think of as fatty, such as pork, contains more protein than fat and its total calorie content may be quite modest. For example, an average portion of rice or pasta may contain 50 g of carbohydrates and around 250 calories in total. That is more than six rashers of grilled bacon (240 calories) and not much less than a generous 125 g serving of roast pork (269 calories).

Fat in our meals is also very useful as it slows down the movement of food through the gut, so that you feel fuller for longer. So it tends to satisfy the hunger, which can mean you actually end up eating less overall. Another advantage of fat is that it does not stimulate the production of insulin, which is, as you know by now, the main fat storage hormone. Fat is, therefore, not fattening just because it is fat. It is only fattening if it is the reason why you are eating too many calories.

Of course, it makes sense not to overindulge in fat, or any other type of food for that matter. However, be careful when buying food that is labelled as 'low fat'. Often it is quite high in sugar. Let us take the example of yoghurt.

Now although zero-fat yoghurt has the fewest calories, it still has the equivalent of nearly two teaspoons of sugar in it – but not much else. It is essentially a thickened sweet drink and is unlikely to satisfy hunger so you may end up eating something else a short time later, cancelling out the benefit of the low calories in the yoghurt.

Table 5: Nutritional content of various yoghurts

	Natural Greek yoghurt	Low-fat flavoured yoghurt	Zero-fat flavoured yoghurt
Sugar (grams per 100 g)	6	13.5	9.3
Fat (grams per 100 g)	9.2	3.2	0.1
Calories	120	98	59

However, if we compare the natural Greek yoghurt with the standard low-fat flavoured yoghurt, you will see that the calorie content is quite similar. Although the low-fat yoghurt has less fat, there is over twice as much sugar (nearly three teaspoonfuls). This will increase the blood glucose level more than the Greek yoghurt and will stimulate the pancreas to produce more insulin to bring it down again. The increased insulin will have two effects – it will stimulate the production of fat, and increase the appetite, again increasing the chance that you will get hungry a short while later.

Although the Greek yoghurt has the highest fat content, this fat is very useful in slowing the absorption of the glucose from the gut, meaning the blood glucose level will rise much more slowly. It also means that you are likely to feel satisfied after a smaller portion, and so the total amount of calories you eat may be less than if you ate one of the other types. As it has the lowest sugar content, the pancreas will release less insulin leading to less fat being stored in the liver and less hunger afterwards.

You could try for yourself eating a portion of each of these three types of yoghurt, checking your blood glucose beforehand and two hours afterwards, and also determining how hungry you feel after two hours. This experiment may help you decide that low fat is not necessarily the best option for someone with type 2 diabetes!

Low-fat foods were introduced in the 1970s as it had been observed that eating a diet that is high in saturated fat was associated with an increase in cholesterol levels. High levels of cholesterol were shown to be associated with increased risk of cardiovascular disease, such as heart attacks and strokes. Many doctors and scientists then linked these two true statements together, to say that – as eating saturated fat increases cholesterol levels, and as high cholesterol levels are associated with increased risk of vascular disease – eating saturated fat must increase the risk of heart disease. This was called the diet–heart hypothesis and led to the recommendation to have a low-fat diet over the past 50 years. However, many more recent studies are questioning this assumption. In 2017, a large study looked at the diets of over 130,000 people in 18 countries and found that there was no association between fat intake and cardiovascular disease. In fact, higher fat intake was associated with reduced risk of death, whereas it was those who had a higher carbohydrate intake who were more likely to die.[22]

Perhaps this provides a clue as to the real associations between diet and heart disease. As we have learnt, a high carbohydrate intake can lead to insulin resistance. It is known that insulin resistance is associated with high cholesterol levels. Insulin resistance is also associated with increased risk of cardiovascular disease. Maybe this was the culprit all along, rather than saturated fat. I do not pretend to be an expert in this area, but as fat is so essential to our bodies, and as obesity and type 2 diabetes numbers have skyrocketed since we moved to a low-fat diet, I do think we should reconsider our approach to fat.

There are several types of fat in our diet (monounsaturated, polyunsaturated (omega-3 and omega-6), saturated and trans fats), and while some are definitely bad, most are now recognized to be very good for us.

- **Monounsaturated fat** is found in olives, seeds and various types of nuts. Nuts have a low carbohydrate content and their fat content (comprising mainly healthy fats) satisfies the appetite – a handful of nuts is therefore a good snack food. The Mediterranean diet is rich in monounsaturated fats and has several health benefits. A major study, published in 2013, demonstrated that eating a Mediterranean diet was associated with a 30 per cent reduction in cardiovascular events (e.g. heart attacks or strokes) compared with a low-fat diet.[23] What is also overlooked or understated is that about half of the fat in meat is also monounsaturated.

- **Polyunsaturated fat** comes in two types. One type is known as omega-3, which is a healthy fat and may help lower the risk of heart disease, depression, dementia and arthritis. Your body can't make it, so it must be in your diet. It is found in oily fish, which ideally should be eaten 2–3 times weekly. (As oily fish can be contaminated with mercury, no more than two portions are advised if you are pregnant, likely to become pregnant or breastfeeding.) Nuts (especially walnuts) and linseed (flaxseed) are also a good source of omega-3. The other type of polyunsaturated fat is omega-6, which is less beneficial. It is found in vegetable oils and spreads containing corn oil or sunflower oil. Too much omega-6 fats can increase inflammation in the body and has been associated with mental health problems.

- **Saturated fat** is found in dairy products and meat. It is also found in coconut and avocado. Recent research has shown that saturated fat is not the enemy once thought and is not associated with increased risk of heart disease. In fact, eating saturated fat is associated with an increase in healthy HDL (high-density lipoprotein) cholesterol levels. In natural foods, it can be considered a healthy fat.

- **Trans fats** are the real baddies. Although they occur in small quantities in some natural foods, such as meat and dairy products, man-made versions are found in many processed foods. They have been shown to increase inflammation and the risk of heart disease. A number of food manufacturers are reducing the use of trans fats (also known as hydrogenated fats) but they can still be found in many baked products and margarines and in foods fried in vegetable oils.

So what about cheese? There is now evidence from a number of research studies that dairy products are not harmful, and some such as yoghurt and cheese may actually be associated with a lower risk of heart disease.[24] Therefore, you can eat cheese. I have lost count of the number of people who express surprise and sometimes shock when I say to them, 'Why not eat some cheese?' They feel liberated after many years of being told not to eat cheese, or to choose low-fat cheese (which can taste like soap). Put simply, I would much rather you ate a small piece of cheese as a snack than a sweet biscuit. Of course, if you eat a lot of cheese, or other dairy products, then you will gain weight. As cheese (like nuts) contains small amounts of carbohydrate, it can be rather moreish and if you are not careful, you can end up eating quite a lot. But a small piece of cheese, preferably without crackers, is a delicious and healthy way to round off a meal. The same goes for butter, which as we learnt in Chapter 6, has just one natural ingredient, and also for unprocessed meat. In summary, dairy products, nuts, seeds, oily fish and meat all contain healthy natural fats and can be enjoyed as part of your eating plan.

CHAPTER 8

Do test your blood glucose levels

Myth: People with type 2 diabetes do not need to check their blood glucose levels.

Fact: Checking your blood glucose levels is invaluable for everyone with type 2 diabetes.

If you have prediabetes, although you are likely to have insulin resistance, your blood glucose levels will often be normal, or only marginally elevated and blood glucose monitoring is usually not recommended. As long as you adhere to the diet principles described in this book and have your HbA1c blood test every few months, then home blood glucose monitoring may not be necessary. That said, if you do wish to monitor your glucose levels, then I would encourage you to follow the advice in this chapter, as recommended for people who have established type 2 diabetes.

The overall aim in managing type 2 diabetes is to maintain blood glucose values that are as near to normal as possible. By definition, to achieve remission requires levels to be no different than in a person without diabetes. If your glucose levels are very high, then you are likely to experience symptoms such as thirst, excessive urination and blurred vision, as discussed in Chapter 2. If your glucose is very low, then you will experience symptoms of hypoglycaemia, which include sweating, shaking and confusion. Between these levels, you may have no symptoms that alert you as to whether your glucose is 4 or 14 mmol/l (70 or 250 mg/dl); you cannot tell what your glucose level is by the way you feel and the only way of knowing your level is by measuring it.

However, in the UK many people with type 2 diabetes are not provided with blood glucose monitoring equipment. It is recognized that glucose monitoring is essential for people who inject insulin, so they can monitor for low glucose levels. It is otherwise not considered essential that people know what their level is! This is a policy with which I completely disagree. Thankfully, things are slowly changing, but many people are provided with no means to measure their blood glucose. This is partly down to cost, as the total bill for glucose testing equipment is very high. But it is also believed that in type 2 diabetes, monitoring does not necessarily help improve glucose control. Furthermore, there was a study performed in Northern Ireland some years ago that suggested that doing regular blood tests was associated with increased depression in people with type 2 diabetes who were being treated with diet or tablets. The problem with that study was that people were asked to check their levels at different times of the day but were not provided with any useful information about what to do with the results. So if your levels are always high and you have no information about how to bring them down, it is easy to see how this might lead to depression.

Since then, a number of other studies have been published that suggest that using blood tests can have positive effects on both diabetes control and wellbeing. The key here is not just blood testing – but structured testing. By that I mean testing in a structured manner in order to provide specific information that can be useful not only in monitoring a person's diabetes, but also in providing specific feedback – which can be very encouraging when the tests suggest that things are moving in the right direction.

From the information provided in Chapters 5 and 6, you will understand that what you eat has a huge impact on your blood glucose levels. I therefore recommend a form of structured testing called paired mealtime testing. This is where you check your blood glucose just before a meal and then two to three hours afterwards. Ideally the glucose level should stay about the same or rise at most by 2–3 mmol/l (30–50 mg/dl). You can use this information to learn to adjust your diet by reducing the carbohydrate in the meal, until the test after the meal ends up within the desired range. For example, if you have a portion of shepherd's pie with some green vegetables, and your glucose increases from 5 mmol/l (90 mg/dl) before the meal to 9 mmol/l (160 mg/dl) afterwards, then it is clear that there was something in the meal that has pushed the glucose level up too high. This is most likely to have been the potato in the pie. So the next time you have shepherd's pie, you could either have a much smaller amount of the potato topping or use mashed celeriac instead, a vegetable that has a much lower carbohydrate content. One you have identified the type and amount of shepherd's pie that enables you to enjoy it without increasing your glucose levels, then as long as you keep to that same amount, you will not need to do a test every time you eat the same meal.

When someone is just starting out using a lower-carbohydrate approach, I generally suggest performing a paired test before and after a different meal each day. For example, breakfast on the first day, lunch the next day, then evening meal and so on. However, it has been shown that just performing a paired test before and after a meal six times a month can help people achieve better control of their diabetes. Using testing in this way does not require a large number of test strips, so need not be very expensive. If you are not prescribed test strips, then they can be purchased online for about £20 (US$30) for 100 strips, which will last a few months.

Using this system means that, once or twice a week, you will be checking your fasting glucose (that is, before breakfast). Even if you do not have breakfast, it is still worth checking your fasting glucose, as it provides a good indication of your metabolic health. You might be surprised to see that your glucose level is quite high first thing in the morning, before you have eaten anything. Quite understandably, people find this puzzling, and wonder where the glucose has come from. The answer of course is that the glucose has entered your bloodstream from your liver. As we discussed in Chapter 2, one of the many functions of the liver is to ensure that you always have enough glucose in your blood, for your body's needs. When you eat, glucose enters your blood from your gut. And if you eat frequently during the day, then the gut will provide your body with all the glucose it needs – and much more. That excess glucose is then stored in the liver as glycogen, ready to be used when extra energy is needed. On the other hand, when we sleep at night, there is a period when there will be no glucose coming from the gut. However, the body still needs glucose to run all its complex processes, and this is where the liver comes in. During the night, the liver begins to use up some of the glycogen stores that it has built up during the day, releasing it as glucose into the blood. All well and good. Except if you have type 2 diabetes.

This release of glucose into the blood from the liver is under the control of insulin. To recap (See Figure 1 on page 24), insulin acts as a tap to turn on and off the flow of glucose from the liver into the blood. If the insulin level is high, the tap is turned off, to keep the glucose in the liver; if the insulin level drops, then the tap turns on, to release glucose into the blood. However, in type 2 diabetes, the liver is resistant to insulin. In other words, the insulin that is present cannot close the tap. It's as if the tap has a leaky washer and glucose continues to drip out from the liver into the blood, all day and all night long. That is why you might have a high glucose level in the morning.

This process can be made worse by what is called the dawn phenomenon. As morning approaches, a whole number of what I call 'wake up' hormones flow into the bloodstream, to gear us up for the day ahead. These include cortisol and growth hormone – and part of the way they work is to make the body even more resistant to insulin, to increase the level of glucose in the blood, to provide us with energy for the day ahead. This dawn phenomenon is completely normal. It just appears to be more marked in some people than others. And it is distinctly unhelpful if you have type 2 diabetes and your body doesn't need that extra sugar rush.

So what can you do about high morning glucose levels? Well, the good news is that as you make dietary changes to reverse your diabetes, two things happen. First, as you eat less carbohydrate, then your meals will not push up your glucose in the first place. And if you make a point of really cutting down on the carbs for your evening meal – and maybe going for a short walk afterwards – you will have done everything you can to end your day with a reasonable glucose level, meaning that even if the liver is leaking glucose during the night, your level the next morning will still be lower than if you had a bowl of pasta the night before. Second, after a while on a low-carbohydrate diet, you will begin to lose some weight and as that happens, your body becomes more sensitive to insulin. That means that the leaky liver tap gets fixed and it will no longer leak glucose into the bloodstream during the night. So, over time, as your body responds to the dietary changes you make, you should see that your glucose levels gradually come down towards normal.

By definition, a normal fasting glucose level (taken first thing in the morning before any food or drink) is less than 6.1 mmol/l (110 mg/dl) and no higher than 7.8 mmol/l (140 mg/dl) after a meal. If you have adopted a low-carbohydrate diet, then levels should be lower than this after meals. A word of advice, however. People who adopt a very low-carbohydrate, ketogenic diet, can find that their fasting glucose is above 6.1 mmol/l (110 mg/dl) and sometimes as high as 7 mmol/l (125 mg/dl) and this naturally causes some concern. This is a recognized phenomenon that is not completely understood. It is as if the body releases glucose in the early morning to prepare for the new day, but the body has adapted to burning fat for its energy and so does not use the glucose, allowing the level in the blood to rise. This is probably a normal physiological response to being 'fat-adapted'. In this situation, I generally say that if your fasting glucose is a bit high, but the level then falls for the rest of the day, and if your HbA1c is within the desired range, then there is no need to be concerned. If, however, your glucose levels stay high during the day and your HbA1c increases, then I would recommend seeking medical advice, as it could indicate that you require medication to manage your diabetes.

Glucose monitoring systems

In the last few years, non-invasive glucose monitoring systems have become available. These systems comprise a sensor, which is usually embedded in an adhesive patch on the skin, with a tiny cannula that sits just below the skin, and a reader, which receives a signal from the sensor and displays the glucose level. There are generally two types: CGM (continuous glucose monitoring), which provides a continuous reading of your glucose level; and isCGM (intermittently scanned continuous glucose monitoring), where the sensor needs to be scanned by a reading device (or using an app in your phone) to obtain a reading. Some systems require a traditional blood glucose reading to be taken once a day to calibrate them and ensure that they are providing accurate readings, while the more modern ones do not. It is important to be aware that these systems measure the glucose in the interstitial fluid, that is the fluid that surrounds the cells in the fat layer beneath the skin, rather than in the blood itself. There is usually a lag time of up to ten minutes between the two. If you are on insulin treatment, then this difference will be more relevant and you will need to be aware that if the sensor is reading low, your actual blood glucose level could already have gone lower; or if the sensor is reading high, the level in the blood could be higher. This difference is rarely an issue in people with type 2 diabetes.

The beauty of these systems is that they mean you can always check your blood glucose at any time of the day and night without the need to do a finger-prick test. They also show you the exact impact of each meal on your glucose levels, and of other activities such as going for a walk. I have no doubt that, in due course and as their costs come down, these will become the standard means of monitoring for everyone with diabetes. At present (2021) in the UK and many other countries, they are not routinely provided for people with type 2 diabetes. Still, the costs are already coming down, and a number of my patients with type 2 diabetes choose to purchase the equipment themselves. At the time of writing, the most widely used system in the UK is the Freestyle Libre system, manufactured by Abbott.[25] The reader (which also doubles up as a blood glucose monitor) costs around £50. Alternatively, you can use an app in your phone to read the sensor. Each sensor also costs £50 ($70) and lasts for two weeks, so the ongoing cost is £100 ($140) per month. It is clearly not cheap but is within reach of many people who do choose to purchase it. Some people use it continually; others choose to use the system for a few weeks at a time. The blood glucose readings can be uploaded into the LibreView system, which allows your designated clinic or doctor to view your data and provide advice on any changes to make in the light of your glucose readings.

There are a number of other systems becoming available and, if using such a system is of interest, I recommend you do your own research online to see what is currently available.

If you do not use a continuous glucose monitor, then it can be helpful to use finger-prick testing to do some intensive monitoring every few months. I recommend doing a seven-point profile. This involves doing a blood test before and after the three main meals of the day and also at bedtime. It has been shown that performing a seven-point profile for three consecutive days once every three months can help people with type 2 diabetes, treated with diet or tablets, to achieve better overall control of their diabetes. It seems that just doing the tests influences behaviour, and often the results are lower for the third day than the first. This is probably because when you see high values on the first day you make changes to your diet – consciously or not. This type of testing has also been shown to increase people's feeling of wellbeing.[26] It is also a good idea to do this more intensive testing for a few days, if your fasting glucose or before-meal blood tests are getting higher, to see if any additional dietary changes should be made.

The aim of home glucose monitoring is to guide day-to-day decisions about food intake and activity levels. Long-term monitoring is done by having an HbA1c check every three to six months. I generally suggest aiming for an HbA1c of around 50–55 mmol/mol (6.8–7.2 per cent) as representing adequate control of diabetes. To achieve remission requires a level of less than 48 mmol/mol (6.5 per cent), through lifestyle changes. Trying to achieve such low levels with certain medications, especially sulfonylureas and insulin, can lead to abnormally low glucose levels without very careful monitoring and adjustment of the medication dose. This is described in more detail in Chapter 13.

Other forms of testing

In Chapter 5, I described how Virta Health in the US encourages a very low-carbohydrate, ketogenic diet that is monitored by measuring ketone levels in the blood. The aim of this intervention is to switch the body to burn fat for energy. Ketones are a by-product of that process and showing that you have raised levels of ketones in the blood (called ketosis) confirms that you are burning fat. I do not routinely recommend measuring ketone levels. This is because many people can get great benefit by reducing their carbohydrates to below 100 g a day, whereas ketosis only occurs when you eat less than 50 g a day. If your aim is to achieve ketosis, then monitoring ketone levels is a way of ensuring that you stay in ketosis. A number of companies make meters that can measure ketones in a drop of blood, using test strips. An ideal ketone level to aim for is between 0.5 and 3 mmol/l.[27]

In Chapter 2, we learnt that in type 2 diabetes, there is not only a problem of elevated blood glucose levels, but that insulin levels are also elevated. In prediabetes, insulin levels are usually elevated to high levels, while glucose levels are still relatively normal. I am often asked, very reasonably, 'Can I measure my insulin levels?' This would seem logical, but insulin tests are quite complex to undertake in the laboratory and are therefore expensive. They are not routinely available in the NHS and many other health systems, but they can usually be performed via a private clinic. In most people with prediabetes or type 2 diabetes, I do not think this is a problem, and as long as the suggested lifestyle changes lead to improvements in body weight, blood glucose and HbA1c levels, then knowing your insulin level is unlikely to make much difference. I will suggest it is measured in cases where there is a doubt as to the diagnosis, and where a person might, for example, have slow onset type 1 diabetes rather than type 2 diabetes. The warning signs for this are where glucose levels remain elevated, or climb even higher, despite making dietary changes, and also excessive weight loss. In this situation, the appropriate tests can be accessed by specialist centres within the NHS.

I am aware from my international work that, in many countries, even basic blood glucose monitoring systems are very expensive and unaffordable. As I described in Chapter 5, I helped set up a project in Nairobi in Kenya, where people on very low incomes attended a programme to help them reverse their type 2 diabetes. They did just as well as their compatriots who attended the same programme in a private hospital across town. They were provided with test strips for the duration of the programme, but otherwise were often not able to afford glucose testing. So, if you are unable to afford glucose test strips, or have an aversion to pricking your finger to draw blood, it is still possible to improve your health and reverse type 2 diabetes without blood glucose monitoring.

Urine glucose testing

Urine glucose testing is a cheaper option but is not recommended. Until the late 1980s, the only method available for a person with diabetes to monitor their diabetic control was by checking the level of glucose in the urine. This involved peeing some urine into a container and dipping a plastic strip with chemicals embedded at one end into the urine. The chemicals reacted with the glucose in the urine, causing the colour of the strip to change according to the amount of glucose in the urine. The colour was then compared with a colour chart to give an indication of how much glucose was present in the urine. Such strips are still available and similar strips are also available to check the level of protein and many other constituents in the urine.

Before the development of these strips in the 1970s, checking the glucose in the urine involved peeing into a container, then adding tablets containing the chemicals and observing the colour change, and before this the technique involved boiling the urine!

Urine test strips are therefore a huge advance on what was previously available. They are cheap and easy to use and, until recently, many people with type 2 diabetes were encouraged to use the method to monitor their diabetes. However, it is very limited in its usefulness for two key reasons:

1. Urine testing relies on the kidneys excreting glucose from the urine when levels in the blood rise too high. However, glucose generally does not appear in the urine until the level in the blood is over 10 mmol/l (180 mg/dl), which is much too high for anyone aiming for good control of their

diabetes. In some people, especially in the elderly, glucose levels can rise even higher before appearing in the urine.

2. Urine is constantly formed by the kidneys and then passes into the bladder where it is stored until a person next urinates, which could be several hours later. Consequently, a urine test is always 'out of date' and does not reflect the level of glucose in the blood at the time the urine is tested.

Furthermore, in the past ten years, a new class of drug has been used very widely, the SGLT2 inhibitors. They reduce the glucose level in the blood by making the kidneys excrete more glucose into the urine, and so anyone taking these drugs will have glucose in their urine; the amount in the urine will no longer reflect the level in the bloodstream, and so they cannot provide any meaningful information about the level in the blood. I therefore do not recommend that anyone uses urine testing to monitor their diabetes.

In summary, if you have type 2 diabetes, I recommend you obtain some means of assessing your glucose control – just not urine testing – as this will be enormously helpful in guiding your food choices, as you make changes to your diet. It is also hugely rewarding and motivating to see levels come down as a result of your efforts. However, it is not absolutely essential, and it is still possible to reverse your diabetes or prediabetes without monitoring your glucose levels.

Our story for this chapter comes from Christine, who used her husband's blood glucose strips to diagnose her diabetes, and then tested her glucose regularly to monitor her progress as she reversed it.

CHRISTINE'S STORY

In March 2021 and at the age of 71 I diagnosed myself with type 2 diabetes. I had been ill for months and, despite several telephone appointments with my GP, the cause of my illness remained undiagnosed. I couldn't stand the smell of food, I felt so sick, but I piled on weight, to around 83 kg (183 pounds). I would often go to bed at 9 pm and would stay in bed until lunchtime, then sleep most of the day in a chair. I could not walk; my legs were like jelly. It was awful. I was breathless all the time and felt useless. Then, after a few months, I started to lose weight. One of the worst aspects was that something was happening to my eyesight: one moment I could see okay, the next I couldn't even make out figures on the TV. I couldn't focus to read, and I stopped driving because I sensed something was wrong. It was very frightening.

I tried to identify the cause of my problems without success and then one day my husband, who has type 1 diabetes, suggested taking my blood glucose reading; it was 27.4 mmol/l (493 mg/dl). By then, I weighed 76 kg (167 pounds). I bought *Reverse Your Diabetes* and started to follow a low-carbohydrate diet. I had to keep it simple, because I was too stressed to cope with a complicated diet. Breakfast was always eggs, lunch was soup or a salad with protein, and evening meals were meat or fish and vegetables. I included nuts and seeds, cream, butter, full-fat milk and full-fat yoghurt. The only fruit I ate was berries.

I kept off bread, potatoes, rice and pasta completely. Originally, I was just going to do it for six weeks, but I found it so easy, and the incentive to reverse diabetes was so immense, that I will hopefully stick to this way of eating for the rest of my life. It was also very encouraging to see my blood sugars reduce so quickly. After just two weeks I had a blood glucose reading of 5.9 mmol/l (106 mg/dl). I was thrilled to see a result so quickly.

I then started to reintroduce some carbs into my diet. I have one Weetabix for breakfast three or four times a week and potato about once a week. I have not touched rice or pasta at all, and only on a couple of occasions had bread. I have 100 ml of red wine three times a week, and one strip of 90 per cent cocoa chocolate each day, as a treat and for medicinal purposes! I would suggest my carb intake is less than 50 g on an average day.

After three months, my weight was 73 kg (161 pounds). My HbA1c level came down from 112 (12.4 per cent) to 45 (6.3 per cent), my cholesterol levels and liver blood tests have also improved. My GP called and said she was astounded that I have achieved so much in just three months. Although I had not lost a lot of weight, it appeared to be shifting as my stomach became quite a bit flatter and my skirts started falling down. My bum disappeared, but I had no idea where the weight was going. I stopped taking omeprazole as I no longer had reflux symptoms. I felt so healthy.

I have achieved this by ignoring the medical advice I was given. One of the nurses was insistent that I could not do anything to change my diagnosis with diet alone, she insisted I should take medication. The recommended diet was carb-based, and if I had followed that advice, I would still be in the same situation I was when I was diagnosed.

When I did the local diabetic course, they hammered home the fact that people with type 2 diabetes are far more likely to suffer strokes, heart attacks, eyesight problems and amputations. They put the fear of God into us. I had to do the course online, so I put myself on mute because what I was doing was so contrary to what I was being told to do. They told us to eat one third of a plate of carbs at every meal and to take the drugs suggested despite the side effects and emphasized we should do as we were told. I didn't dare make any comment.

Blood testing was key to helping me regain my health. Although the NHS does not recommend it (or provide testing kits to people with type 2 diabetes), I started testing my blood four times a day. I kept meticulous records of everything I ate, all my blood sugar readings, how I felt, even when I went to the loo. If I introduced something new, for example one roast potato with my Sunday lunch, I tested my blood before I ate it and then two hours after to make sure there were no adverse reactions.

I used *Reverse Your Diabetes* as a guide. I followed the principles but adapted the philosophy to suit my own lifestyle. I have found this new way of eating remarkably easy, and far preferable to yet more pills. I was told years ago, 'If God didn't make it don't eat it', but unfortunately, He did not tell me to exclude bread, pasta and rice!

I have no longer got a burning, painful liver, I no longer have reflux, I no longer have bile malabsorption, my cholesterol readings have improved without medication and, for the first time in over 20 years, I do not have diarrhoea almost every day. It sounds daft but it is fantastic to be going to the toilet properly once again. I am sleeping well, no more disturbed nights with reflux. No more wetting myself, which was very, very embarrassing. No more chronic fatigue and most importantly my eyesight has returned to normal. Now I feel alive again.

All this has been done with a low-carb diet. I have not been able to exercise because I have a hernia which has been a problem recently, and I refused to take any medication. I just cannot understand how such a simple change to one's diet can promote such beneficial changes. It's truly unbelievable, and as I said my doctor couldn't believe what I had achieved in such a short time.

———————————————————————

CHAPTER 9

Exercise is not the answer

Myth: You need to exercise to lose weight.

Fact: Exercise is not the answer. Just walk more and sit less.

For many years, exercise has been recommended for people with diabetes because it has been shown that it helps reduce blood glucose levels. However, the evidence suggests that it does not have a big impact. Regular aerobic exercise, such as running or 'cardiovascular' workouts, has been shown to reduce HbA1c by around 8 mmol/mol (0.7 per cent), and anaerobic or resistance exercise (such as weight training) by around 6 mmol/mol (0.5 per cent). Combining the two does slightly better, resulting in a 9 mmol/mol (0.8 per cent) improvement. However, to achieve these improvements it is estimated that it is necessary to exercise for at least 150 minutes per week; anything less than this will make little difference. In many studies, where the amount of exercise achieved was measured, the average was only around 60 minutes a week. Good for many aspects of health, but not enough to have a meaningful impact on blood glucose levels.

I see so many people in clinics who, when they realize that their weight has gone up, or their glucose levels are high, respond with,

'I know I need to exercise more.' For many years now, we have all been exhorted to exercise. The official guidance for all of us is to do 150 minutes of moderately intense exercise every week – that means enough to make you a bit breathless and sweaty (or as the NHS website politely puts it, 'make you breathe faster and feel warmer'). Their list of ideas for exercise includes brisk walking, water aerobics, riding a bike, dancing, doubles tennis, pushing a lawn mower, hiking and rollerblading.[28] Arguably, the only ones that are widely accessible are brisk walking and riding a bike (but only if you own one). Both, however, can be a challenge for someone who is overweight, has joint pains, foot problems or a heart condition – all of which are more common in a person with type 2 diabetes. For many people, it can seem like the official advice sets them up to fail, and if they are unable to achieve the recommended level of exercise, it can lead to a sense of despondency, demotivation and even failure, especially if their weight and/or glucose levels continue to go up.

If this is familiar to you, then I have what I hope will be welcome advice – ignore the guidelines. For so many in our society, I just do not think they are fit for purpose.

So far in this book, we have focused on the dietary changes that will help you control, and hopefully reverse, your prediabetes or type 2 diabetes. There is a good reason for that: they are the changes that really will help you lose harmful excess fat and achieve better health. Exercise is great for your heart and for building muscle strength. It is also great for mental health and wellbeing. But it is not great for losing weight or controlling diabetes. The studies show that it only has a small effect. In fact, anaerobic or very high intensity exercise can actually increase blood glucose levels and so can be counterproductive. For people who are very overweight, exercise can pose a real risk of injury. That's why I say, exercise is not the answer.

Walk more

For some years now, I have not used the word 'exercise' in this context. For too many people, it is associated with negative connotations – of failure, of pain, of the dreaded Lycra, of having to go to a gym, of embarrassment about body image in the changing room, and so the list goes on. People are usually very happy when I say don't exercise. Instead, I recommend that they walk. Not a brisk walk, just a walk, or more accurately movement. I recognize that some people are unable to walk and so any movement or physical activity will do.

Some of the earliest evidence for the benefit of walking came from research in the 1950s that looked at the health of two groups of workers in London: bus drivers (who spent several hours sitting behind the steering wheel) and bus conductors, whose job was to sell tickets to passengers, moving along the rows of seats and up and down the stairs at the back of double-decker buses all day long. The study also looked at postal workers, who spent much of their day walking delivering mail, and telephone switchboard operators who, like the bus drivers, were seated during their working hours. They found that the more active workers (postal workers and bus conductors) had lower death rates from heart disease than their less active colleagues.[29] The negative effects of being less active were demonstrated in a study from Denmark, in which active healthy volunteers were persuaded to reduce their activity from over 10,000 steps a day to less than 1,500. After just two weeks, they had already demonstrated evidence of higher blood insulin levels and a significant increase in abdominal fat.[30]

In the 1950s, many more people were physically active at work than now, when so many of us work at a desk all day. However, we can make up for this by how we get to work. Researchers looked at the health of over 20,000 people from the UK who took part in a national survey and described how they got to work. Any type of 'active travel' to work (walking, cycling or using public transport) was associated with a lower likelihood of being overweight.[31] Walking and cycling to work were both associated with a lower likelihood of having diabetes. However, the message is that you don't have to walk or cycle all the way to work to benefit. As most people using public transport have to walk to and from the bus stop or train station each day, using a bus or train is actually better for you than driving.

I had my own experience of this when, many years ago, I worked at a hospital in London. I had to walk to my local station to catch the train and, after a 30-minute train journey, walk from London's Waterloo Station to the hospital. In total, I was walking nearly 3 miles (5 kilometres) every day. I then moved jobs to a hospital where I had to drive for 90 minutes each day to get to work. At a stroke, this increased my sedentary time by 2 hours and reduced my exercise time by 50 minutes every working day. Guess what happened – my weight began to increase.

Over the past ten years, there has been a gradual trend towards people spending some of their time working from home. This became the norm for many more people during the lockdowns of 2020 and 2021, when we were all instructed to stay at home, thus removing the physical activity associated with getting to and from work. So, for people who work from home, I still encourage them to 'walk to work'. By that I don't mean just walking from the bedroom to wherever your computer is (and for some people that might not even require getting out of bed), but before you start your work, and when you finish, go for a 20-minute walk.

Not only will it help reduce your glucose levels, but it will also increase your wellbeing and brain function and hopefully make the day more enjoyable or productive as a result.

Walking is the ideal physical activity. It is free and does not require any special equipment, and it's also a very useful form of transport. Unless you are predominantly based at home, I do not focus on going out for a walk, as that requires making the time to fit a walk into your routine. Rather, I encourage everyone to build walking into their daily routine. By this, I mean making it an automatic part of your day. This can be achieved in the following ways:

- If travelling by bus, get off at least one stop before you need to, so that you have to walk part of your journey.
- If driving somewhere, find a place to park a few hundred metres from where you need to be.
- If shopping at a supermarket or other store with a large car park, park as far away from the store entrance as you can.
- Choose to walk or cycle rather than use a car for any trips less than 1.5–2 km (1–1.5 miles).
- Use stairs rather than elevators or escalators.

If you are not used to walking, then I recommend you choose one or two of these changes and give them a try. Remember, you do not have to walk briskly; any walking speed is better than not walking. If you are overweight, then your knees or hips may ache to start with. But as you lose weight, these aches and pains should ease. The more you walk, the more your strength will improve and the easier you will find it. You might actually enjoy it.

There are many reasons why walking is pleasurable. A 20-minute walk significantly increases brain activity and with it a feeling of wellbeing. Research has shown that being in green spaces improves health and wellbeing. That doesn't have to mean a walk in the country, it could be in a town park or along a riverbank, so if you can include these on your walking route to work or to the shop, then you will have added benefit.

Sit less

My first message around physical activity is to walk more; the second is to sit down less, or more specifically to try to avoid sitting for longer than one hour at a time. So many of us spend several hours each day, whether at work or at home, sitting in front of a screen, be it a TV screen or a computer. Again, this is a huge change from just a few decades ago. Anyone over the age of 50 will remember when in the UK there was no TV until mid-afternoon, and even then there was only a choice of three TV channels. They will also recall typewriters – mechanical machines where pressing letters on a keyboard caused each letter to be printed onto a piece of paper, one by one in real time. They were made obsolete by the arrival of computers. Anyone over 40 will remember a time when most homes did not have a computer, and anyone over 30 will remember a time when a mobile phone just made phone calls. These technological changes to our environment mean that, for many of us, work, play, shopping and socializing can all be done from the sofa, where we can spend hours on end, sitting, slouching or lying down. This is called sedentary time and it is bad for our health.

A lot of research has examined the impact of sedentary time. In one study, over 500 adults with newly diagnosed type 2 diabetes were asked to wear an accelerometer, a wearable device that measures activity levels. They also had various other measurements performed to assess their overall metabolic health. The accelerometers were analysed to determine how long they were inactive. The study concluded that the longer the sedentary time each day, the greater the level of insulin in the blood and the worse the insulin resistance. This inactive time was also associated with an increase in waist circumference of nearly 2 cm (about ¾ of an inch), and with a reduction in healthy HDL (high-density lipoprotein) cholesterol – both known consequences of insulin resistance.[32] So, it is possible that the more time we spend sitting down, the more likely we are to develop type 2 diabetes. Indeed, this was the conclusion of a meta-analysis of a number of studies that looked at the effect of time spent watching TV on people's health. This showed that, on average, for every two hours spent watching television each day, the risk of developing type 2 diabetes increased by 20 per cent, and the risk of death from all causes increased by 13 per cent. Incredibly, people who spent five hours a day watching television had a 50 per cent increased risk of developing diabetes. Of course, it may not just be the sitting down which is bad for your health; unhealthy food eaten while watching television may also contribute. Also, another way of looking at it is to argue that, in some cases, people are watching too much television because they are overweight and less mobile in the first place. Nevertheless, even taking these factors into account, the research suggested that two hours a day watching television was associated with a 13 per cent increased risk of type 2 diabetes.[33]

You may think that doing the recommended 150 minutes of exercise a week would mean spending less time in front of the television. Well, it isn't necessarily the case. A study in Australia looked at data from over 4,000 people who all did at least 150 minutes of moderate to vigorous exercise each week. They were asked how long they spent watching television, and it was found that even in this 'healthy' group, spending longer in front of the television was associated with a bigger waist circumference, higher blood pressure and higher blood glucose levels.[34] The authors of this study described such people as 'active couch potatoes'! This type of study is very important as it emphasizes that the good that comes from exercise can be undone by too much sitting down.

Even if one doesn't watch television, modern life means that long periods of sedentary time are inevitable for many people – for example, those whose job involves driving or sitting at a desk. What can these people do to try to preserve their health? Studies have looked at the effect of 'breaks' in sedentary time. The study I mentioned earlier of the 500 people who wore accelerometers showed that those who interrupted their sedentary time, even for just one minute, had a smaller waist circumference. This was confirmed in another study that showed that having more breaks during sedentary time was associated with a reduction in waist circumference, body weight and blood glucose levels, compared with subjects who did not interrupt their time sitting down.

There are a number of possible reasons for this, including the fact that the act of standing, even for a short time, uses significantly more energy than sitting down. I explain it using an analogy with a computer. If you do not use your computer for a certain amount of time, it goes into sleep mode. That is, it is still on, but the screen has switched off and the processors have stopped whirring, in order to conserve energy. In the same way, if we do not use our body for a period of time, our metabolism goes into a sort of sleep mode, and slows down to use just enough energy to keep things ticking over. As a result, blood glucose levels rise and the energy saved is stored as fat in the liver, hence the increased waist circumference. The simple act of standing up has a similar effect to moving your computer's mouse – it wakes the machine up and it starts operating again at full speed, consuming more energy as it does.

My second piece of advice regarding activity is therefore to try to avoid sitting down for longer than an hour. That means that if you are sitting at work all day, at your desk or in a meeting, or in front of the TV at home, try to make it a habit to stand up at least once an hour and walk around for a couple of minutes, before sitting down again and continuing with what you were doing. You do not even have to leave the room, although if you did venture outside for a couple of minutes, that would boost your system in other ways too. Many people set their watch or their phone to buzz every hour to remind them. At work, I suggest people try to make their office as 'inefficient' as possible, so that the printer or filing cabinet are not right next to their desk. Better still, use a standing desk or an adjustable height desk so that you can work while standing.

Sitting in front of a screen can cause other problems too. For many years, I experienced pain in the back of my neck. Then, a couple of years ago, I developed a lot of pain in my left shoulder. It was diagnosed as impingement syndrome (which I had never heard of) and I was told that it was due to my age. My GP advised that I might need steroid injections or even surgery to correct it but suggested we try physiotherapy first. I saw a really good physiotherapist who said it was mostly due to bad posture, especially spending long periods of time sitting at a desk, and that with exercises and a better posture, I shouldn't need injections or surgery. Perhaps to prove to myself that this wasn't a problem of my age, I diligently did the exercises he recommended and converted an old square high table into a raised desk. I used that exclusively in my home office for several months and – lo and behold – the shoulder recovered completely. I then gradually reverted to the comfort of my sitting desk, until a few weeks ago, when the other shoulder developed the same problem – so I am again, right now, standing at my table.

Previously, when I heard about people using standing desks, I used to think, surely their legs would ache, surely it must be tiring. Every so often I use a stool to rest my legs while using the raised desk but mostly I can work for a whole day while standing, giving me a much better posture, and relieving symptoms that otherwise might have required surgery. Is there a similar change that you can make to reduce the time you spend sitting down? It might not only help improve your glucose levels, it might also help improve shoulder and neck pain!

Another problem from too much screen time is eye strain. After several long stints of writing this book, using my standing desk, I began to experience eye strain and headaches. My eye test was overdue, so I went to my optometrist for an eye check and was asked, 'Don't you know about the 20-20-20 rule?' I said I did not. Essentially, anyone who spends long stints in front of a computer is advised to pause every 20 minutes, for just 20 seconds, and to focus on something 20 feet (6 metres) away. I don't think this last 20 has to be exact but moving away from your computer and looking outside the window or walking into another room will ensure you do what is needed – move your focus away from the near-distance of the screen. If you walk away, you will presumably need to get out of your chair if you are seated and so the 20-20-20 routine will not only protect your eyes, but also avoid the dangers of extended sedentary time.

Being more adventurous

So many people are delighted when I say to them: don't exercise, don't even think of joining a gym – just walk more and sit less. However, as they then lose weight, as they find they can walk further without aching or getting short of breath, and especially as they feel healthier and better about themselves, many people then choose to be more adventurous. They might get out an old bike and rediscover how much they enjoyed cycling. They might feel confident enough to join a local parkrun, safe in the knowledge that it is okay to walk, or to stop and start. Parkrun is an initiative started in 2004 in Bushy Park in outer London, the local park of my childhood, right behind my parents' bakery. It is a weekly, organized event with a 5-km (3-mile) marshalled circuit that has since spread to hundreds of locations in over 20 countries. As the organization's website states, it is weekly, free, 5 k, for everyone, forever.[35] The 'for everyone' means that, sure, there will be some who do the 5-km circuit at breakneck speed, but it is not a race. The whole point is that it is a safe environment for anyone to enjoy exercising – on their own, or with a group of friends. Some walk all or part of the 5 km, others push children in buggies or run with dogs on a lead. The 'forever' has had to be interrupted due to lockdowns, but the aim is that, in normal times, it will always be there, reliably every week and therefore be as accessible and available as possible.

Other initiatives include the Couch to 5k app, which provides a structured programme of gradually increasing activity over nine weeks, taking a person from total inactivity to running 5 km. For people who yearn to play football again, there is Walking Football, created to enable people to enjoy the game they used to love playing, but at walking pace.

If none of these take your fancy, you may enjoy a longer walk or cycle ride in the countryside or maybe getting a dog who needs a walk every day. There are many rainy, windswept days when my wife and I are out with our dog, and we think no one in their right mind would be out in this weather – except for those who have to walk their dog.

Right now, participating in any kind of exercise may just seem too much to contemplate. That's absolutely fine. However, please do consider what changes you can make to walk more and sit less. And when you feel motivated to do something more energetic, maybe have another look at this chapter.

Chris's story illustrates how being a regular runner did not protect him from developing type 2 diabetes – but changing his diet did. Once he had reversed his diabetes, his running improved no end!

CHRIS'S STORY

I am 47 years old and live in Yorkshire in the north of England. I work as an adviser to businesses in financial distress: it is a challenging job, involving a fair amount of stress, and often long working hours. Despite being a keen runner, over the years my lifestyle took its toll. In the years leading up to my diagnosis of type 2 diabetes, I started to gain weight, developed fatty liver and high blood pressure. I was more susceptible to infections and had a lot of dental problems. I had annual medicals where the advice was to eat a low-fat diet, which I tried and failed at. No one mentioned diabetes or insulin resistance.

Then in May 2018, aged 44, I was told I had type 2 diabetes. I weighed 102 kg (225 pounds) and my HbA1c was 66 (8.2 per cent). The doctor offered me a consultation with a dietitian but also helpfully scribbled down a reference to diabetes.co.uk. He also sent me a blood monitor (finger prick) and a few strips.

My initial reaction was shock: I had never heard anyone say the words out loud, 'I have type 2 diabetes.' There was so much stigma and I was afraid. I looked up the consequences, the complications: amputations, heart attacks, strokes. I thought about my father, who died of a heart attack aged 49. I'd spent years angry and confused about his death, blaming his smoking. Maybe he also had undiagnosed diabetes.

Over the following ten days I did my research and went to the diabetes.co.uk forum and headed straight for the success stories section: the very fact it existed made me excited. My doctor had said the disease was 'inevitably progressive' and 'a slope, and our job is to slow the rate you slide down the slope'. Now I was reading that this could be reversed.

I watched Dr Sarah Hallberg's TedTalk on reversing diabetes, I read Dr David Cavan's *Reverse Your Diabetes* and Gretchen Becker's book *The First Year: Type 2 Diabetes: An Essential Guide for the Newly Diagnosed*, and, based on all the success stories I'd read, I built a plan. I was now a low carber. I didn't dive in full cold turkey, but migrated over about three weeks.

Week one, breakfast became eggs; week two, I tackled dinner, introducing substitutes for starchy carbs; week three, I focused on my work lunch – tinned sardines, mackerel, sliced meat, hard-boiled eggs. No more sandwiches. The finger prick testing was a key part of learning what foods did to my blood glucose.

Within eight weeks, I was on the very low-carb, keto diet that I now follow. More importantly within eight weeks I was in remission. My HbA1C was down to 40 (5.8 per cent). After 12 weeks I had lost about 20 kg (44 pounds) in weight. All my blood tests improved, apart from my LDL (low-density lipoprotein) cholesterol level. My doctor could only say, 'Wow.' Mostly it was easy. I missed some things, especially toast, crumpets with jam, and Yorkshire puddings. But on the whole the results I was getting, especially the weight loss, were enough motivation for me.

Having reversed my diabetes, I was ready to go public. People had noticed the weight loss and were making comments. At first, friends and colleagues were shocked, but incredibly supportive and interested in what I had achieved. Quite a few felt challenged and were not ready to accept some of the central messages of what excess ultra-processed food does. But numerous contacts approached me on behalf of themselves or loved ones, to seek guidance and access to resources to help them too.

Being able to help others fix themselves is hugely motivational and probably the best aspect of the journey. But for me, adopting a low-carb lifestyle and reversing my diabetes has given me back a sense of energy, purpose and enjoyment that was dwindling before.

I began to enjoy my running again. I'd been getting slower and slower in the years leading up to 2018. Then having lost the weight, I was quickly doing more than one 10-km (6-mile) run a week. One morning I got up and ran and ran and (a bit like Forrest Gump!) just kept going; within 2 hours I'd done my first half marathon in 20 years (my wife rang me, to check I was okay). Then in 2019 I ran my first ever marathon, and also my first ever ultra-marathon – 50 km (31 miles) along the canals of Lancashire and Yorkshire (all before breakfast). At the finish I was elated. Probably my greatest physical achievement ever. My experience shows that even if you run regularly, that doesn't stop you developing diabetes if you also have a bad diet. Fixing the diet fixed my diabetes – and enabled me to run much better than ever before!

In short, I was on a collision course with an early death, just like my dad. But with the help of the right advice, and the right support, I got onto the path to better fitness than most of my adult life… and I've met some wonderful, supportive people along the way who I now count as firm friends.

_____

CHAPTER 10

You do not need to eat breakfast

Myth: You must eat three meals a day.
Fact: You don't need to eat if you are not hungry – missing meals can be good for you.

Let me start with a question. Why do you eat breakfast? This is a question that I have increasingly asked patients in recent years, as I am genuinely interested in the answer. Why? Because it appears that, for many people, breakfast is a chore. They don't actually enjoy it. Often, they are not even hungry. So, why do they eat it? Many people feel they should, largely because they have been told, 'Breakfast is the most important meal of the day' or 'You must have your tablets in the morning with food', and especially once they developed diabetes, 'It is important to eat regular meals.' Indeed, the NHS website says that people with type 2 diabetes should 'eat breakfast, lunch and dinner every day – do not skip meals'. Some websites even recommend people with diabetes should eat six small meals a day.

Now it is true that, many years ago, people whose diabetes was treated with insulin were advised to have three main meals, plus snacks mid-morning, mid-afternoon and at bedtime. The reason for this was that they were on one or two injections of insulin each day, at a fixed dose. There was no means of checking their blood glucose levels, and the insulins used were, by today's standards, quite primitive and were absorbed at different rates on different days. So, to minimize the risk that their blood glucose would fall too low, they were advised to eat regularly during the day, and you guessed it, all meals should contain some carbohydrate (although in those days the amount of carbohydrate was restricted and standardized every day). This notion of needing to eat regularly has remained within the diabetes world ever since, even though we now have the ability to manage diabetes with many medications that do not risk low glucose levels, and glucose levels can be measured continually if so desired. It is almost as if parts of the diabetes establishment are stuck in the 1960s with their advice. I genuinely cannot think of any other area of medicine where there is such a hangover in practice from so long ago.

As a result, many people with type 2 diabetes, who are overweight and therefore need to eat less, often feel obliged to eat even though they are not hungry. I have lost count of the number of people who have told me that they never used to eat breakfast until they were diagnosed with diabetes. Some people sheepishly tell me that they don't eat breakfast and then think I will tell them off. They are usually mightily surprised and relieved when I say it's fine. In fact, as I then go on to explain, missing breakfast, far from being harmful, could be doing them a lot of good. Not just because it means they are not eating unnecessary food that will make it difficult for them to lose weight, but also because there is now a lot of evidence for the beneficial effects of what is called intermittent fasting.

Intermittent fasting first hit the headlines about ten years ago, when Dr Michael Mosley introduced us to the concept of the 5:2 diet, in his book *The Fast Diet*. Until then, I associated fasting with religious practice, most obviously among Muslims who fast during daylight hours during the month of Ramadan. Fasting is also practised by many other faith groups, with claims that it helps cleanse the body and/or the spirit. It's fair to say that I was sceptical that fasting conferred any real benefits to physical health. In his book, Dr Mosley opened my eyes to the different ways in which fasting is beneficial to our physical health. One is that the body uses periods of fasting to undergo essential maintenance; fasting increases a process called autophagy, which literally means self-eating, i.e. the body rids itself of ageing and decaying cells. He also lists many other benefits to longevity, to the heart and the brain. But the most striking impact of fasting is on the level of insulin in the bloodstream. While many health professionals share my previous scepticism about intermittent fasting, in 2019 the prestigious medical journal, *The New England Journal of Medicine*, published an article promoting the benefits of intermittent fasting and time-restricted eating.[36]

We learnt in Chapter 2 that insulin levels increase when we eat a meal that contains carbohydrates, and that high insulin levels over time lead to excessive accumulation of fat in the liver and the pancreas, and this drives the development of type 2 diabetes. Reducing carbohydrates reduces the insulin levels in the blood, but protein, and to a lesser extent fat, also leads to some insulin being produced. In some people, this may be enough to stop them losing weight. However, when we fast, insulin levels fall really dramatically. That is because there is no longer a steady stream of energy coming from our food, and so the body needs to access its stored energy. The first stores to be used are the glycogen (glucose) stores in the liver and muscles, which, when insulin levels fall, are released into the blood. These are soon used up, and so then the fat stored in the liver is used as energy. This release of fat stores out of the liver is halted as soon as insulin levels rise again. Therefore, when we fast, insulin levels remain low, and the longer that we fast, the longer our insulin levels remain low and the more fat stores will be used up. Fasting is therefore remarkably effective at removing excess fat, and much cheaper than liposuction. The 5:2 diet is an approach whereby you eat normally for five days each week, but on two days, you 'fast'. Well, you don't fast completely, you are allowed one meal of about 500 calories. Michael Mosley used this approach to reverse his type 2 diabetes, and many others have also found it successful.

But what about breakfast? Well, missing breakfast is another great way of fasting, and arguably easier as you don't need to do any special planning for it – you just get up and go each morning, skipping breakfast. This essentially creates a 16-hour fast each day. You can have an early lunch and an evening meal no later than 7 pm; you can even have a mid-afternoon snack if you wish. But then you eat nothing from 7 pm until at least 11 am the next day. This is a relatively short fast, but studies have shown, in both mice and humans, that even if you eat the same amount of calories each day, restricting your eating to this eight-hour window is associated with less weight gain and lower insulin levels. Some people are happy to miss breakfast every day, others feel hungry on some mornings but skip breakfast on days when they do not.

So, if you do not like breakfast, or are often not hungry in the morning, try skipping it. If you take tablets with breakfast, speak to your doctor about what to do if you miss breakfast. Some can be taken on an empty stomach; those that need to be taken with food can generally be taken at lunchtime.

There are other forms of intermittent fasting that are a bit more involved. I generally do not recommend these to people at the outset of their journey to reverse their diabetes or prediabetes as I encourage the focus to be on changing what to eat, rather than when, in the first instance. But, for people who need to lose a lot of weight, or when weight loss has stalled, I will suggest they try introducing fasting. If they are still having breakfast, the first stage would be to miss breakfast for a few days each week. The next stage would be to have two 24-hour fasts each week. This is a variation on the 5:2 approach, but means that on a fasting day, you miss both breakfast and lunch, so you just eat an evening meal. Some people routinely have just one meal each day (also called the OMAD approach) and feel perfectly well doing so. Others prefer to do a 36-hour fast a couple of times a week, where on fast days you miss all meals. It is important to drink plenty of plain fluids when you fast. This can include tea and coffee with a small amount of milk or cream. Some doctors recommend a cup of broth, or low-calorie soup, on fast days, to provide some salt and other minerals.

You might think you couldn't possibly manage to miss one meal, let alone a whole day of meals, as you constantly feel so hungry. The reality is that many people report they rarely feel hunger when they fast, and if they do, it soon passes, especially if they do something to take their mind off it. The reason is that hunger is to a large extent driven by insulin, and if you are used to eating carbohydrates several times a day, you are keeping your blood insulin levels up quite high, so that you always feel hungry. Remember that, during a fast, insulin levels and also hunger are greatly reduced.

As I mentioned earlier, fasting for health reasons is a new concept to me, but both the theory and the results I have seen have convinced me that it can be extremely useful. However, I felt I owed it to my patients to at least have tried it myself. A couple of years ago I started to skip breakfast, not every day, but on some days when I knew I was going to be busy (I had been advised that fasting is easier when you have a lot to do – and less time to think about food). Most days I found I didn't really feel hungry in the mornings, but if I did, I would have breakfast, which for me is usually plain Greek yoghurt with berries and some seeds. I also found that my two cups of coffee each morning kept my stomach from rumbling, and I could easily last until lunchtime without eating. I then extended my fast on some days by missing lunch – I would just go out for a walk instead. On some days, particularly when working in clinics, I found it less easy to concentrate by mid-afternoon. On other days, when I had more free time, I found that I could fast until the evening by going out for a longer walk or cycle ride during the afternoon. Indeed, I recall one occasion when I was in Bermuda and decided to do a 24-hour fast by missing breakfast and lunch. Having worked all morning, I went off for a bike ride in the early afternoon. Bermuda is only about 20 miles (30 kilometres) long and I would often ride a circuit to one end of the island and back. Parts of the island are quite hilly, with some steep climbs that require a lot of leg work. But on this particular day, I found it almost effortless – the climbs seemed much easier than usual. Then I recalled stories of people who undertake really quite intensive exercise while fasting and find that they perform so much better than when loaded with carbs. This is because if you exercise while fasting, your muscles can adapt to burning fat for fuel that can lead to enhanced endurance. I am not an expert in this area, but this very unscientific personal experiment certainly seemed to show that fasting added a certain something to my cycling that I had not experienced before.

Fasting is not for everyone and there is no one right way to do it, but if you wish to explore using fasting as part of your routine, I encourage you to find a routine that works well for you. It is essential to discuss with your doctor any changes to your medication that might be needed, particularly if you take insulin or sulfonylurea tablets, or other tablets that need to be taken with food. Dr Jason Fung, a kidney specialist from Canada, is a leading expert on fasting, and his book *The Complete Guide to Fasting* provides a wealth of information on the practicalities of introducing it into your routine.

If, for whatever reason, you do not feel that fasting is for you, then I encourage you to use the evidence of its benefits and only to eat if you are hungry. Please, ignore the instruction that you must not skip a meal. If on a particular day you get to lunchtime and you are really not hungry, then don't eat lunch. Or if you had a late and large lunch so that you are not hungry in the evening, don't eat again in the evening. If you meet a friend for coffee, remember that the coffee will fill your stomach and you really don't need to have something to eat with it. It is highly unlikely that our prehistoric ancestors sat down in the caves to eat three meals a day. In fact, the mechanisms that we have evolved to store excess energy as fat suggest the opposite. These fat deposits are a safety net, built up during periods of abundance for the lean times when there is no food available. The trouble is that for far too many of us there is always too much food (or highly processed products that masquerade as food) available – all feast and no famine. The more we can get back to a pattern of only eating when we are hungry, the more our bodies will be able to function in better metabolic health.

MARIA'S STORY

I was born in 1966 in Lincolnshire in England. I have had weight issues all my life and was put on my first low-fat diet at nine years of age. After the birth of my son, I developed severe migraines that got progressively worse and one time I ended up in hospital with stroke-like symptoms. I was given a leaflet which suggested I control my blood sugar levels. At the time, the Atkins diet was popular and so, after a lot of research, I started a low-carb diet in September 2002. I lost 19 kg (42 pounds) in weight and had no more migraines. I stayed on less than 25 g of carbohydrate a day, which kept me free from migraines, but over the next 14 years my weight crept up again.

In 2017, work was stressful and in July I slipped and pulled my back. It seemed to take a long time to recover and then I started to wake in the night with pain under my shoulder blades. Once awake, I needed the loo. I was taking naps in the day to make up for lack of sleep at night. I'd developed word blindness, struggled to think of the words I wanted to say and mispronounced a lot of them. I developed bladder urgency and high blood pressure. In October 2017, my doctor arranged some blood tests and my HbA1c came back at 87 (10.1 per cent). I had developed type 2 diabetes even though I was on a low-carb diet.

I was prescribed metformin, a statin and a blood pressure tablet, and the diabetic nurse told me I would be on pills for life. She said diabetes wasn't reversible, gave me a snack sheet with suggestions such as toasted tea cake, mashed banana and maple syrup... Having done Atkins for 15 years, I knew this was TOXIC for a diabetic. I went home and looked for more support on the internet and found the Diet Doctor website and social media groups for ketogenic diets.

I didn't have to reduce carbs any further, but I reduced my protein intake and increased my fats. I took just one metformin a day (not the four prescribed) and I bought my own blood glucose testing equipment as in the UK these are not prescribed for people with type 2 diabetes. After three months, my HbA1c was 50 (6.7 per cent). My doctor was sceptical, but supportive and told me to stop taking the metformin.

After another three months, my HbA1c was 42 (6.0 per cent). My doctor told me it was okay to be prediabetic. I told him it wasn't! After one year, I had lost 25 kg (55 pounds) and my HbA1c was 31 (5 per cent). My doctor stood up, shook my hand and said he thought I was a model patient. The new diabetic nurse was more receptive to low-carb diets and asked me questions about it.

At my second anniversary, my HbA1c was 30 (4.9 per cent) but I had barely lost any more weight.

I had already reduced my protein intake and couldn't go much lower, so I looked towards extended fasting. I already did intermittent fasting, eating within a 4–5-hour window each day. I started alternate day fasting in February 2019.

Due to Covid, my annual check was delayed to November 2020. By then, my HbA1c had reduced to 28 (4.7 per cent) and I'd lost another 8 kg (18 pounds), my lowest weight since my mid-teens. My cholesterol level improved too.

It has been difficult to stick with alternate day fasting and a change of jobs did not help (the constant need to explain why you're not eating). I've tried to keep to one meal a day (OMAD or 24-hour fasting) with a longer fast at the weekend if my social calendar allows. As I've been low-carb for a long time, I don't really miss foods, but I have learnt many alternatives such as keto bread and celeriac for potatoes and pasta. I try not to have too many sweet treats; I save them for when eating with friends and they think I miss out without a dessert. So, I always make one to take and share.

As well as reversing my diabetes and losing weight, my diabetic retinopathy has resolved. I no longer struggle to find the words I need or mispronounce them, have no more bladder urgency and no more naps. I can also walk much more than previously.

I now know that I'm very hyperinsulinemic (high insulin levels in the blood) and that is why I needed to reduce protein as well as carbs to lose weight. However, I have learnt that fasting is the key to keeping my insulin low for as long as possible to enable me to keep the weight and HbA1c down.

_____

PART THREE

Helping you on your way

CHAPTER 11

Step by step towards your new way of eating

Having read the last few chapters and busted a few myths, I hope you feel motivated, even excited, to begin to make some changes that will set you on the path towards reversing your diabetes or prediabetes. Let's summarise what we have covered. Diabetes or prediabetes is not your fault. It can be reversed, and to do so, you will need to make some changes to what and when you eat. It also helps to move more and sit less.

In this chapter, I am going to focus on some of the practical steps you can take to start off on your journey to a healthier future. But first of all, I would like you to revisit the goal-setting questions we introduced in Chapter 1:

1. What frustrates you most about your health at present?

2. How do you want things to be different?

3. How will you feel when you have achieved this?

4. What is your main goal – the thing you would like to achieve from reading this book?

Have a look back at the answers you wrote for Chapter 1 (on page 10 or in your notebook) and have a think about whether you want to change any of them after reading the subsequent chapters. If so, write out your new answers on these pages or in your notebook, and bear them in mind as you read this chapter. I will then suggest you try to break your main goal down into smaller 'bite-size' changes you can begin to make to start you off on your journey – or to take you to the next stage, if you have already made some of the changes suggested in Chapter 1.

We have explained that the most important changes you can make to help you reverse the diabetes disease process and improve your health are changes to your diet, specifically reducing your intake of sugary and starchy foods and drinks. One approach is to go 'cold turkey' and stop all foods and drinks containing sugar and starch in one go. This is advocated by some clinics and is necessary for anyone wanting to reverse their condition by using a very low-calorie diet. If you feel you can do this, then the advice that follows will still apply and you will need to make all the changes at once. You will need to have your diabetes medications reviewed to ensure that you do not run into any problems once you change your diet – further information about this is provided in Chapter 13.

Many people prefer to make changes more gradually, and in the following pages I will suggest a step-by-step approach to reducing your intake of carbohydrates. Hopefully, you will then get an idea of what changes you think you can make to start off with, ones that you think you will be able to sustain, before moving on to other changes. Do bear in mind though, that if you feel you have addictive feelings towards certain foods, then these will have to be stopped altogether at some stage if you want to avoid these foods controlling your eating. This is discussed in more detail in Chapter 12.

Step 1: Stop sugary drinks

Probably the most important first step is to reduce your sugar intake. I think there is enough evidence of the harm of sugar-sweetened beverages to suggest that the priority here is to cut out all sugary drinks. These include the obvious – such as cola and other types of fizzy drink – but also the less obvious, including fruit juices, smoothies and sweetened hot drinks. The same applies to some of the flavoured cappuccinos available in popular coffee shops. Take a look at Table 6 (overleaf).

Fruit smoothies have been marketed as very healthy, and there are now all sorts of gadgets and pre-prepared mixes of frozen fruits available so you can make them at home. We have already discussed how some fruits are not a healthy option if you have diabetes, but all fruits, when turned into a smoothie, become a very sweet drink, albeit with some fibre in it. As you can see from Table 6, in terms of sugar they are on a par with Coca-Cola. Sure, the sugar is 'natural' in as much as it originally came from a fruit, but it is still sugar, and will have a big impact on the level of glucose, and therefore insulin, in the bloodstream. For this reason, I suggest avoiding fruit juices and smoothies, alongside all manufactured sugary drinks and flavoured hot drinks sweetened with any type of sugar, syrup or honey. In Table 6, I have listed the grams of sugar per 100 ml of each drink, and then the amount of in a 'typical serving'. I have then calculated the rough equivalent in a typical serving as teaspoons of sugar.

Table 6: Sugar content of popular drinks

Drinks	Grams of sugar per 100 ml	Serving size	Grams of sugar per serving	Teaspoons of sugar equivalent per serving
Flavoured cappuccino*	10.9	300 ml mug	37	9
Coca-Cola	10.6	330 ml can	35	9
Hot chocolate*	9	300 ml mug	27	7
Fruit smoothie	Up to 11.0	200 ml glass	22	5.5
Orange juice	10.5	200 ml glass**	21	5
Cranberry juice	5.8	200 ml glass	11	3
Cappuccino*	3.6	300 ml mug	10	2.5
Milk (whole)	4.7	200 ml glass	9.4	2
Tomato juice	4.3	200 ml glass	9	2
Coffee / Tea (dash milk) (black)	0.5 0	300 ml mug	1.5 0	Less than 0.5 0
Almond milk (unsweetened)	0	200 ml glass	0	0
Water	0		0	0

Source: All information derived from the Tesco UK website in May 2021, apart from items marked * which are from the Starbucks website.

** A serving of fruit juice is often shown as 150 ml, but that is a very small glass.

There are not many things that I suggest avoiding completely, but sweet drinks are one of them. I would go so far as to say that I do not think it will be possible for a person to reverse prediabetes or type 2 diabetes if they continue to drink sugar in this way. If you do like sugary drinks, please consider switching to diet versions that use artificial sweeteners as a first step in reducing your sugar intake. Sweeteners can also cause problems – for example, by prompting cravings for sweet things – but they are a much less bad option than sugar, and a good way of weaning yourself off sugar. Ideally, I suggest you eventually aim to limit your intake of artificial sweeteners as well.

From this information, you can see that to minimize liquid sugar intake, the best drinks are water or unsweetened tea or coffee. If you crave sweetness, by all means use an artificial sweetener; you can also add a slice of fruit or cucumber to add flavour to a glass of water, whilst unsweetened herbal teas are another good option.

Step 2: Reduce snacking

The next stage is to cut right down on the sugar you eat. Many natural foods have small amounts of sugar, so it is not possible to avoid it completely. Removing foods with added sugar, however, is essential. As discussed in Chapter 6, that means cutting right down on confectionery, biscuits, cakes, ice cream and desserts, as well as sweet fruit. A lot of these foods are snacks rather than part of our main meals. So, rather than focusing on a long list of foods that you now need to avoid, I encourage you to think of it another way – by cutting out snacks.

Snacks are an invention of the food industry, and they pour hundreds of millions of pounds into developing and advertising them to us. Whereas in the past, parents would tell children not to snack as it will 'spoil your appetite', now the all-pervasive messaging that comes through marketing encourages everyone to get through tonnes and tonnes of snacks, many of which are ultra-processed and high in sugar. So, I encourage you to focus on eating enough at your main meals to fill you up, and then aim to avoid any food between meals. That means having your mid-morning cup of tea or coffee on its own, without a biscuit, a banana or bar of chocolate (or if you are in a coffee shop – a cake or pastry). If we are honest, we do not need any of these additional foods; we eat them because we like them and quite often because it has become a habit. We may enjoy the first few mouthfuls and the sugar rush, but then feel rather bloated and uncomfortable afterwards. Try going without a snack, and you will find that you can still enjoy your drink – and as it fills your stomach it will give you a feeling of satiety, without feeling that you have overdone it.

If you tend to fill up on biscuits, chocolate or cake between meals, then avoiding these will automatically reduce your sugar intake very significantly. By reducing your blood glucose levels, this will also reduce your insulin levels, which means you will likely feel less hungry between meals – so there will be less desire to snack. Also, remember that reducing insulin levels is key to reversing the diabetes disease process.

There will be times when you feel peckish – so it is important to ensure that you have some healthier snacks available to you. Examples include a small piece of cheese, a few strawberries, some vegetable sticks, a handful of nuts, a hard-boiled egg or a piece of dark chocolate. Note that, while a small handful of raisins or a plain biscuit are also low in total carbohydrate, their sugar content may make you crave more and, despite your best intentions, you could end up eating more than you intended. For this reason, I suggest avoiding sweet snacks wherever and whenever possible.

Table 7, and all the following tables, show the grams of carbohydrate (sugar and starch) per 100 g of each food, and then the amount of carbohydrate in a 'typical serving', as well as the rough equivalent of the carbohydrate in a typical serving given in teaspoons of sugar.

Table 7: Carbohydrate content of popular snacks

Snacks	Grams of carbo-hydrate per 100 g	Serving size	Grams of carbo-hydrate per serving	Teaspoons of sugar equivalent per serving
Iced bun	59	116 g	69	17
Mars bar	69	51 g	35	9
Pain au chocolat	42.5	75 g	32	8
Banana	23	200 g	30	7.5
Fruit scone	55	38 g	21	5
Croissant	44	40 g	16	4
Wholemeal toast	38	40 g (slice)	15	4
Packet of crisps	53	25 g	13	3
Chocolate biscuit	66	15 g	10	2.5
Raisins	66	15 g (handful)	10	2.5
Small apple	11	85 g	10	2.5
Carrot sticks	7.4	100 g	7.4	2
70% dark chocolate	36	20 g	6	1.5
Rice cake	77	7 g	5.6	1.5
Satsuma	6	85 g	5	1
Cracker	68	8 g	5	1
Plain biscuit	71	7 g	5	1
Strawberries	6	85 g (6–7)	5	1
Mixed nuts	8	25 g (handful)	2	0.5
Celery sticks	1	100 g	1	0.25
Cheddar cheese	0.1	30 g	Trace	0
Hard-boiled egg	Trace	30 g	Trace	0

Note: All information derived from the Tesco UK website in May 2021.

Maybe you do not eat cakes or biscuits, but you enjoy eating fruit – perhaps five or more pieces a day. You can be forgiven for thinking you are doing the right thing, as all the official diet messages encourage us to eat fruit. However, some fruit – such as bananas, pineapple and mangoes – are very high in sugar and best avoided, unless you can eat just a very small portion. A single grape is low in carbohydrate, and as long as you eat no more than five at a time, this should be fine. If you find stopping at five difficult, then they too are best avoided. I generally suggest getting your five a day from vegetables rather than fruit. However, if you do wish to have fruit, remember 'berries are best', followed by a small apple, plum or tangerine, or really any fruit that you can easily fit in the palm of your hand. Remember that dried fruit is very high in sugar, and so prunes, raisins, dried apricots and other dried fruit are best avoided.

I know that, for some people, cutting out all sugary snacks will not be easy. Whether you recognize that you have a sugar addiction or a sweet tooth, or you just really enjoy eating sweet treats, you might find it difficult to cut out all sugary foods completely. If that is the case, then start by identifying one or two small changes that you think you can make. It could be having one instead of two biscuits, cutting down on orange juice or trying a sweetener in your tea instead of sugar. It could be having an apple instead of a pastry. It does not really matter what the change is, so long as it is one that you think you have a reasonable chance of achieving. However, if you feel genuinely addicted to certain foods, the aim should be to stop them completely, as we will discuss in Chapter 12.

Step 3: Reduce starch in breakfast

For many people, reducing their sugar intake will have a big effect in improving their glucose levels, which is great. Many others will have cut out a lot of sugary foods when they developed type 2 diabetes or prediabetes. However, they may also be consuming a lot of starchy foods – this, after all, was the advice they received. Remember that starch is just sugar molecules holding hands, and just like sugar, it increases the glucose and insulin levels in the blood. Reducing starchy foods is therefore an essential part of reversing the disease process.

For Step 3, I suggest focusing on breakfast. There are three main reasons for this. Firstly, an easy way to reduce starch intake is simply not to have breakfast; secondly, when I ask people what they eat for breakfast, a huge majority say that they have starch in the form of cereal and/or toast. Thirdly, breakfast time is the worst possible time to challenge the body with carbohydrates. At this time, the levels of many hormones such as cortisol and growth hormone are quite high. These 'wake up' hormones prepare the body for the day ahead – and part of the way they work is to counter the effect of insulin to keep your blood glucose level high. That means, if you have diabetes or prediabetes, insulin resistance is worse at breakfast time than at any other time of the day.

Table 8 (overleaf) lists some of the common foods we eat for breakfast. As I have said, for many of us, breakfast means having a breakfast cereal. It was my standard breakfast for years and years.

Table 8: Carbohydrate content of popular breakfast foods

Breakfast foods	Grams of carbohydrate per 100 g	Serving size	Grams of carbo-hydrate per serving	Teaspoons of sugar equivalent per serving
Just Right cereal	79	40 g	32	8
No added sugar muesli	63	40 g	28	7
Fruit'n Fibre cereal	67.4	40 g	27	7
Weetabix	69	40 g (2 Weetabix)	26	6
Coco Pops cereal	84	30 g	25	6
Cornflakes	84	30 g	25	6
Porridge	60	40 g	24	6
Bran flakes	65	30 g	19.5	5
White bread	46	40 g (medium slice)	19	5
Wholemeal bread	38	40 g (medium slice)	15	4
Fruit yoghurt pot	11.6	14 g	14	3
Plain Greek yoghurt	5.3	100 g (2 dsp)	5.3	1.3
Mixed berries	5.7	35 g (1 dsp)	2	0.5
Tomato	3	80 g (1)	2	0.5
Mushroom	0.3	80 g (3–4)	0.2	0
Egg	Trace	30 g	Trace	0
Bacon	Trace	30 g	Trace	0

Note: All information derived from the Tesco UK website in May 2021.

I knew, of course, that very sugary cereals like Coco Pops, shamelessly marketed at children, were not healthy, but somehow I was convinced that the grown-up alternatives, such as porridge or muesli, were much healthier. But are they? From Table 8, you can see that a standard serving of 'no added sugar' muesli has more carbohydrate than Coco Pops!

Next, look at bread. A typical slice of bread is 15–20 g of carbohydrate. If, like many of my patients, you have a bowl of cereal and a couple of slices of toast, this could easily add up to 80 or 90 g of carbohydrate, in just one meal, at a time of day when your body is least able to deal with it.

The most important advice I can provide regarding breakfast is to stop eating breakfast cereals – all of them, including the 'healthy' ones. Unless you really enjoy a particular cereal and can limit yourself to a very small portion – like Christine, whose story we read at the end of Chapter 8, who allows herself one Weetabix a few days each week. At 13 g of carbohydrate, that is consistent with a low-carb diet – but only if she sticks to a single Weetabix with a small amount of milk! Plain (full-fat) Greek yoghurt with some mixed berries is a natural, filling and healthier alternative, with a fraction of the carbohydrate content. If you have time to cook, then eggs and bacon, or a mushroom omelette will fill you up with practically zero carbs!

Finally, the most zero-carb option, of course, is to skip breakfast, as part of a time-restricted eating regime, as we discussed in Chapter 10. Unlike what many of us have been told for many years, missing breakfast can be positively good for you. Are you willing to give it a try, maybe once a week?

Step 4: Have a low-carb lunch

Just as breakfast can add up to a huge carb load, so can lunch – or what has become a usual lunch for many of us. A sandwich, packet of crisps and a piece of fruit can easily total nearly 70 g of carbohydrate – see Table 9 (overleaf) for common lunch choices.

Table 9: Carbohydrate content of popular lunch options

Lunch foods	Grams of carbohydrate per 100 g	Serving size	Grams of carbohydrate per serving	Teaspoons of sugar equivalent per serving
Baguette (white)*	25	230 g	58	14
Sandwich (wholemeal)*	38	80 g (2 slices)	30	7.5
Wrap*	60	50 g (small)	30	7.5
Tomato soup (tinned)	6.8	300 g	20	5
Mixed bean salad	12.5	125 g	15	4
Green vegetable soup	4.8	300 g	15	4
Chicken soup	4.9	300 g	15	4
Tomato soup (fresh)	4.7	300 g	14	3.5
Tuna salad	2.5	300 g	7.5	2
Sardines (tinned)	Trace	120 g	Trace	0

Notes: All information derived from the Tesco UK website in May 2021.

* The table shows the carbohydrate in the bread/wrap alone. Any carbohydrate in the filling will be extra.

I have been asked if a wrap is a better option than a sandwich and the answer is no, as a wrap can easily contain the same, if not more, carbohydrate than two slices of bread. I am also asked if crackers or crispbread are better than bread. From Table 7 on snacks (page 187), you would have seen that again, the answer is no, unless you can limit it to one or two crackers. Although they are small, crackers are basically concentrated flour and therefore very high in carbohydrate. The *Carbs & Cals* app and books are extremely useful resources to help you understand how many carbs are in different types of food.[37]

A low-carb lunch really needs to move away from flour-based foods. My general advice is to have soup or salad. As you can see in the table, a salad has very few carbs, and if you choose carefully, many soups are also low carb, especially if you make them yourself. Home-made soup, especially vegetable soup, is remarkably easy to make, and in my experience is usually (bar a few mishaps) rather delicious. You can make up a large quantity and take it to work in a container to microwave, or in an insulated flask. For salads, I generally say use whatever you would have put in your sandwich, but with some lettuce and tomato instead of bread. Add a hard-boiled egg or a handful of nuts and you have a high protein (and therefore very filling) low-carb lunch.

Another lunch alternative is a tin of sardines. A lot of people have not opened a tin of sardines for many years. They associate them with their childhood and for some the experience has kept them away ever since. I quite liked sardines as a child, and until recently I always thought of them as a child's meal. However, even though my children have long since left home, we do have them in the house now that I have realized how healthy they are; my wife and I sometimes share a tin of sardines to have with salad for lunch.

A couple of years ago, one of my patients said they took a tin of sardines to work for lunch. It might not be as easy to eat as a sandwich, and you probably shouldn't try it while walking around town, but with a bit of care, you can eat sardines from the tin at your desk. They are packed full of protein and healthy fats with near-zero carbohydrate. So, a few weeks ago, I tried it myself. I dared not take a tin to work so one day, when working at home, I had a tin of sardines for lunch – and nothing else. In fact, they are so densely packed with nutrition that I could only manage to eat three of the four sardines in the tin. The dog enjoyed number four. They kept me full right into the evening. In the UK at least, they are also very cheap, at around 40 pence for a 125-g tin of sardines in olive oil or brine. Much cheaper than any shop-bought sandwich or 'meal deal'.

There are some situations where it is very difficult to avoid eating a sandwich for lunch, especially at a work meeting or as a guest. In this situation, I suggest eating the sandwiches with the thickest fillings – eat as few as you need to, in order to feel satiated, and if you think you can get away with it, leave the crusts. As a scientific experiment, I made a really thick egg salad sandwich at home, with two 40-g slices of wholemeal bread. I ate the middle part with all the filling and deliberately left the crusts and the corners that had no filling and weighed the remnants. They totalled 20 g, or fully a quarter of the total weight of the bread. This reduced my carbohydrate intake from 30 to 22 g for that meal.

I have written many times about my relationship with bread that stems from growing up as a baker's son and having freshly baked, warm, crusty bread in the house every day. My bread intake is now a fraction of what it used to be, but it is something I really enjoy. As do many of my patients, especially if they bake their own. The good news is that there are some low-carbohydrate breads available. One is Burgen bread, which has around 12 g of carbohydrate per slice; lower-carb Hovis has less than 10 g per slice. There are also low-carb alternatives to flour, which you can use to make very passable bread.

Step 5: Think 'meat and two veg'

When it comes to main meals, my simple advice is to think of 'meat and two veg' type meals rather than meals based on potatoes, pasta or rice. Perhaps, more accurately, 'protein and as many veg as you can manage' would be a better description – one that includes meals for non-meat eaters and encourages you to pile your plate up with as many veg as you like. So, any type of meat, poultry, fish, seafood, pulses, nuts, seeds, cheese or eggs, prepared in any way you choose, together with an array of fresh or frozen vegetables. The only considerations to be aware of are to avoid flour-based sauces and to be mindful that root vegetables contain starch. Even so, you can occasionally add a few small new potatoes or chips, if you really cannot manage without them. It's as simple as that!

From Table 10 (overleaf), you can see that the way potatoes are cooked affects their carbohydrate content. Boiled potatoes absorb water, thus reducing the carbohydrate in a given weight, whereas roasting or frying dehydrates them and makes the carbohydrate more concentrated.

Pasta and rice are also high in carbohydrate and can push up your blood glucose to a really quite high level. If you enjoy meals with pasta or rice, you can adapt them to use vegetable alternatives. For lovers of takeaway curries, you can still enjoy many of the dishes, although beware that some may contain sugar. Instead of having them with rice, try curried mixed vegetables, or even a base of shredded lettuce. We have trained our minds and stomachs to believe that curries have to be served with rice or chapattis. They don't! Some people create cauliflower rice by stir-frying grated cauliflower. Personally, I prefer the texture of whole cauliflower florets, but if having something that looks like rice helps your mind to accept it better, then so be it. Instead of pasta, invest in a spiralizer to create courgette (zucchini) spaghetti to enjoy with your Bolognese. And instead of mashed potato on your shepherd's pie, try mashed celeriac or cauliflower, with just a fraction of the carbohydrate found in potato.

Table 10: Carbohydrate content of popular starch options
in main meals

Starches in main meals	Grams of carbohydrate per 100 g (cooked)	Serving size	Grams of carbo-hydrate per serving	Teaspoons of sugar equivalent per serving
Chips/fries	30	150 g	50	12.5
Roast potatoes	26	150 g	40	10
Baked potato	21	150 g	32	8
Mashed potato	16	150 g	24	6
Boiled potatoes	15	150 g	22	5.5
Sweet potato	17	100 g	17	4
Pasta	33	150 g	50	12.5
Basmati rice	30	150 g	45	11
Couscous	25	150 g	37	9
Wild rice	21	150 g	32	8
Parsnips	12.5	100 g	12.5	3
Carrots	8	100 g	8	2
Celeriac	2.3	100 g	2.3	0.5

Note: All information derived from the Carbs & Cals website in May 2021.

If you wish to reduce your carbohydrate intake to very low levels, then you will need to take into account the carbohydrates in vegetables. For this purpose, I find it helpful to consider vegetables in four broad categories: salad vegetables; leafy vegetables; legumes (peas and beans); and root vegetables.

Salad vegetables, such as tomatoes, cucumber, and red and green peppers, are in fact the fruits of the plant as they contain the seeds. However, they are generally eaten as vegetables. They all have quite low sugar content and can be eaten freely.

Leafy vegetables are generally from plants where we eat the green leaves that grow above ground. Examples include broccoli, cabbage, spinach, lettuce and cauliflower. These are all rich in fibre and vitamin C, with very low sugar or starch content, and can be eaten in unlimited quantities.

Legumes are a class of vegetable that produces beans that are either eaten alone, such as pulses, peas or broad beans, or together with their 'pods', such as French beans, runner beans or sugar snap peas. Their carbohydrate content varies considerably and so it is important to know which ones are high and which are low in carbohydrate. Any that are eaten with their pods are low in carbohydrate and can be eaten freely. Split peas and chickpeas contain about 40 per cent and 50 per cent carbohydrate respectively, and are best avoided as they are often eaten in quite large quantities. Lentils and black-eyed beans are better options, but still contain around 20 per cent carbohydrate; red kidney beans are only 7 per cent carbohydrate.

Garden peas are relatively low in carbohydrate. However, beware mushy peas – which are very dense and can contain much more carbohydrate than you might think. Sweetcorn is strictly speaking a grain but is often viewed as a vegetable similar to peas. However, its name is a bit of a giveaway as it contains around 20 per cent carbohydrate, and anything more than a very small portion will increase your glucose level.

Root vegetables are those where we eat the roots, such as all types of potatoes, carrots, turnips, parsnips and beetroots. These roots store energy for the plant, which helps them to survive as they lie dormant over winter. Much of this energy is in the form of starchy carbohydrate and for this reason anyone with diabetes should eat root vegetables in moderation. Some, such as onions, carrots and swedes are about 10 per cent carbohydrate, so a usual portion will contain very little carbohydrate. Potatoes and parsnips are higher and should only be eaten in small quantities. Beetroot is 10 per cent carbohydrate, of which 7 per cent is sugar.

When it comes to desserts, I generally suggest trying to manage without them, as if you eat a good main meal, your body won't need a dessert. But if you do fancy a dessert, then berries with full-fat Greek yoghurt, crème fraîche or double (heavy) cream are all very tasty low-carb options. If you are having a special meal, then there are some low-carb desserts in the recipe section of this book (see page 358). Emma Porter at thelowcarbkitchen.co.uk shows how you can also make a delicious chocolate mousse with coconut milk or whipped cream and 90 per cent dark chocolate. She also has recipes for low-carb crackers if you prefer cheese after a meal. Alternatively, eat cheese with celery instead of crackers.

Step 6: Watch what you drink

We have already covered the need to reduce sugar in soft drinks and hot drinks. But what about alcohol? The good news is that alcohol is no more or less harmful for a person with type 2 diabetes or prediabetes than a person without, and the recommendations are the same – to limit consumption to 14 units a week or less. Like fructose, alcohol is very efficient at filling the liver up with fat, which as we have learnt is one of the key issues in the diabetes disease process. Alcohol is also very high in calories. Therefore, if you wish to lose weight, and especially if you drink in excess of 14 units a week, reducing your intake will certainly help. Some people choose to stop drinking alcohol altogether for a while as part of their journey to reverse their diabetes.

If you do drink alcohol, then it is important to know what effect your drinks will have on your blood glucose levels. As alcohol is produced by fermentation of sugar, then as a rough rule of thumb, the higher the alcohol content, the lower the sugar content, as shown in Table 11.

Table 11: Carbohydrate content of popular alcoholic drinks

Alcoholic drinks (% alcohol by volume)	Standard serving size	Grams of carbohydrate	Units of alcohol
Smirnoff Ice (5%)	275 ml bottle	25–30	1½
Low-alcohol beer (less than 1%)	330 ml bottle	20	trace
Low-alcohol wine (less than 1%)	175 ml (regular) glass	20	trace
Cider (5%)	1 pint	20	2½
Liqueur (Baileys Irish Cream, Tia Maria) (17–20%)	50 ml glass	15	1
Stout (Guinness) (4%)	1 pint	15	2
Beer (3–4%)	1 pint	10	2
Lager (5%)	330 ml bottle	10	2
White wine (12.5%)	175 ml (regular) glass	5	2
Red wine (15%)	250 ml (large) glass	5	4
Port, sherry, vermouth (15–20%)	50 ml glass	5	1
Vodka (40%) with slimline mixer	25 ml (single)	0	1
Gin or Bacardi (40%) with slimline mixer	50 ml (double)	0	2
Cognac (40%)	50 ml (double)	0	2

Source: Bournemouth Diabetes and Endocrine Centre.

Most spirits have no sugar in them. Red wine or dry white wine has a low sugar content and should not adversely affect your glucose levels, especially if drunk with a meal. Beers contain carbohydrate and so I generally advise beer drinkers to consider beer as any other carb-containing food and avoid it as much as possible. The worst offenders are cider, sweet liqueurs, 'alcopops' and low-alcohol wines and beers, which are best avoided.

Alcohol can affect the liver's ability to release glucose into the bloodstream and this can lead to excessively low blood glucose levels in heavy drinkers. This is rarely a problem in people with type 2 diabetes, unless they are on treatment with medication, such as insulin or sulfonylurea tablets that increase blood insulin levels.

Low carb for people on restrictive diets

Anyone who is on a restricted diet for health reasons, such as gluten or lactose intolerance, will need to ensure that, as they make changes to their diet, they do not inadvertently introduce a food that they should avoid. As low carb generally means reducing wheat products, then this is unlikely to be a problem for people with gluten intolerance. Many people increase their intake of dairy products, such as butter, cream and cheese, and although some people with lactose intolerance can tolerate some of these products, they should be vigilant when trying new foods, or seek lactose-free alternatives.

Vegetarian and vegan diets are usually high in grains (such as rice and quinoa) and flour-based foods, as well as legumes as they provide plant-based sources of protein. They are, of course, also high in carbohydrate and so these will need to be reduced in order to follow a low-carb diet. It is therefore essential that adequate protein is consumed from other sources. For vegetarians who eat eggs and dairy products, this will not be so much of a problem, as these provide sufficient protein. For vegans who choose not to eat any animal products, it is important to be aware of the need for adequate plant sources of proteins. These include nuts, seeds and soy-based products, such as tofu. Even a low-carb vegan diet is likely to include some legumes (beans, peas, lentils), and so a very low-carb, ketogenic diet might be difficult to maintain for a vegan. Nevertheless, it should be possible to maintain a carbohydrate intake of less than 100 g per day on a vegan diet, which for some people will be sufficient to fully or partially reverse their type 2 diabetes or prediabetes. A word of caution though. In recent years, many new 'fake' meat and dairy products have been produced, aimed at vegans and vegetarians. By definition, these are ultra-processed foods, which as we learnt in Chapter 6 are really not foods at all, but chemical compositions designed to maximize sensory pleasure from eating, shelf life and profitability. They come with their own health risks and I generally recommend that these are best avoided. The Diet Doctor website (www.dietdoctor.com) provides excellent advice and recipes using real foods for vegetarians and vegans who wish to adopt a low-carbohydrate diet.

Having identified your main goal at the start of this chapter, please take a minute or two to think about what specific changes you feel you can make, and when you will implement them. Maybe start by looking at the tables in this chapter to see if you can switch from some of the high-carbohydrate choices to lower-carb alternatives. In the next chapter, we will explore how to make a start with changes and how to stick with them.

SHASHIKANT'S STORY

I am from Mumbai, India and I work for a pharmaceutical company. I was diagnosed with type 2 diabetes in 2015, when I was 48. I was previously diagnosed with fatty liver and had acid reflux symptoms and joint pains. Otherwise, I felt in reasonably good health but my weight was increasing gradually.

When I was diagnosed, I weighed 69 kg (152 pounds) and my HbA1c was 55 (7.2 per cent). I received no specific advice except to cut down on rice, sugar and potatoes, to eat wheat instead and to follow a low-fat diet. I started to search the net for a solution and came across www.dlife.in, which is a low-carb community in India. I became convinced that this was the solution for diabetes. I am a vegetarian and eat dairy products. I added eggs and focused on eating more protein foods. I started to change one meal at a time, and over a period of time slowly changed all my meals. I now eat two meals a day instead of three.

It was difficult to get off the rice-based Indian diet and I missed my favourite Indian snacks and also chocolate. So, I started making zero-sugar chocolate at home. I felt under pressure from my family who questioned what I was doing and discouraged me almost daily, but I managed to stay on track. I kept my carbs to under 50 g per day and lost 10 kg (22 pounds) in weight. My HbA1c came down to 32

(5.1 per cent). I look better with a flat tummy and no longer experience hunger pangs or acid reflux. My joint pains also improved significantly and overall I feel more confident in myself.

....

CHAPTER 12

Making changes and sticking to them

If you have read this book from the beginning, there is a good chance that you have already made some changes to your diet or other aspects of your daily life. Or maybe you are actively considering making some changes in the next few weeks. If you still do not feel ready to make changes, it might be better to wait until you do feel ready before committing to change – that way, you are more likely to keep going with the changes.

There is absolutely nothing wrong with not being ready to make changes. It is human nature that we all do the things that we think are important for us right now. If, at the moment, you do not think it is important to make a change, then it's probably not worth trying; you will be setting yourself up to fail. That isn't the same thing as saying you do not understand how a change may be beneficial to your health; rather it is an acknowledgment that there is something else in your current circumstances, which might include a family or work situation that is consuming all of your energy, that is more important to you right now.

The key is always – are you ready to change? In order for you to assess this, it might be helpful to ask yourself two questions:

1. On a scale of zero (not at all important) to ten (extremely important), how important is it for me to make changes to help reverse my type 2 diabetes or prediabetes?

2. On a scale of zero (not at all confident) to ten (extremely confident), how confident do I feel that I can make those changes?

When I ask my patients those questions, many give a high score in answer to the first question. After all, they have chosen to come to see me to discuss their health. However, the answers to the second question often vary quite a lot. If your answer to both questions is high, then you are ready to change. However, if your answer to the second question is four or five, then you should follow it up with some further questions:

1. Why did I score so low for the second question?

2. What would need to happen for me to be able to give myself a higher score?

This may prompt you to focus on any barriers you have to making the changes to your lifestyle, so you can address those barriers and be in a better position to make the changes. Let me give a personal example. When I was at school, I was never any good at sports. I have memories, from a very young age, of being the last to be picked for a team in football; being placed at the back where I would cause the least damage and standing there in the freezing cold for much of the game. I remember being so cold that in the changing room afterwards, my fingers were too numb for me to be able to do up my shirt buttons. My relationship with any kind of organized physical activity went downhill from then on and stayed with me into adulthood. I did, however, love cycling, but that stopped when our children came along and family life took over. Fast-forward 15 years and I entered my forties a few pounds heavier than ideal and doing no exercise at all. A friend suggested we go for a cycle ride. It was tough terrain but I felt so unfit that at times I was gasping for breath. I realized I needed to improve my fitness and considered joining a gym, but my early unpleasant experiences came flooding back and were enough to stop me from doing anything about it. I recognized that as the source of the barrier, but wasn't motivated to do anything to overcome it. Then, a couple of years later, my brother challenged me to join him in taking on the Three Peaks Challenge. This involves climbing the highest peaks in England, Scotland and Wales within a 24-hour period. Crazy. There was no way I could achieve that without some serious training, and that meant joining a gym to strengthen my muscles and increase my exercise capacity. Suddenly, the need to prove to my younger brother that I could rise to his challenge overcame the barriers that had held me back over the previous years. I joined the gym, got fit and nine months later completed the challenge in 23 and a half hours!

Looking back, this is a good example of how setting a goal, however crazy and apparently unrealistic, can be motivating enough to prompt you to make significant changes to achieve it.

In Chapter 11, I invited you to reaffirm your main goal and to think about some changes you could make to help you achieve it. But how realistic are those changes? On a piece of paper, write down the changes that you feel you can make in order to achieve your goal. Alongside each one, write the scores to the two 'readiness to change' questions – how important is it and how confident am I – and then add them up and put them in the final column. You will end up with something like this.

My goal is: To lose weight.

In order to do this, I will aim to make the following changes:

Change	How important is it for me to do it? (0–10 scale)	How confident am I that I can do it? (0–10 scale)	Sum of both scores
Stop drinking fruit juice	10	10	20
Walk round the block each evening	10	6	16
Stop snacking	7	3	10
Use a standing desk	7	6	13
Stop eating breakfast cereals	8	6	14
Eat less bread	8	7	15
Eat more vegetables	9	8	17

In theory, the change with the highest score is the one that you will find easiest to do followed by the one with the next highest score. So, in this example, the first thing to do will be to throw away (or give away) all the fruit juice you have in the house. Now this may be less easy if you live with someone who craves fruit juice every day, in which case you may need to manage your change in a less drastic way, but the point is you need to do something to show you and those around you how determined you are. Then, make sure you have enough vegetables in the house to fulfil your next planned change of eating more vegetables. Then, set yourself a reminder to go out for a walk after your evening meal, before you get settled down in front of the TV. It may be helpful to write down your top three changes, and how you will achieve them – and, very importantly, when. You may feel there is never a good time to make changes. It may be that you have an important event, such as a holiday coming up, or a wedding to attend, or a job interview. If so, it is reasonable to wait until that has passed before making changes. But if not, and now that you are actively contemplating making changes, there is nothing like starting now, today.

Change	How will I achieve this?	When will I start?
Stop drinking fruit juice	Stop buying it; tell everyone I no longer drink it	Today
Walk round the block each evening	Go after evening meal	Next week
Eat more vegetables	Buy frozen green beans, and fresh cabbage	Today

Once you have achieved these changes, then you can consider addressing the next item on your list and so on. You don't necessarily have to go through this process with every change you plan to make, but it may be helpful to start with. The aim is that you only plan to make changes that are SMART. That is:

- **Specific** – so you know exactly what you are going to do.
- **Measurable** – you know how to tell if you have achieved it.
- **Achievable** – it has to be a change that you are able to make.
- **Realistic** – and one which you have a realistic chance of making.
- **Timely** – and one for which you can specify a time of making it.

Please note that the changes I have used in this example are just examples. You have to be honest in choosing the ones that are the SMARTest ones for you.

Make a food plan

By now, you will have an idea about the changes you want to make to help you achieve your goal. Having decided which foods to eat, and which to avoid, it helps to write out a food plan, or at least a list of what you will have for breakfast, lunch, evening meal and snacks.

Over the years, many people have asked me for a food plan. This is because they have been on countless diets with varying success and are used to being told what to eat – that is, after all, what dieting is about. Eat this and eat that, don't eat the other. But why delegate such a fundamentally important question to someone else? Our food is what nourishes us and builds or destroys our bodies and brains. You are now taking an interest in understanding and deciding which foods you want to eat for the sake of your own health. So – don't ask for a food plan. Now that you know what changes are likely to be helpful for you, and what foods you like to eat, make your own plan. Where possible, eat real natural foods the way nature intended (real meat, fish, vegetables, eggs, dairy, natural unprocessed fats) and avoid processed foods and drinks as much as you can. If you decide to keep some in your diet, consider whether you can use them as a temporary measure that you will eventually replace with the real, natural equivalent. Remember, fats are not inherently bad and so don't be afraid of natural, unprocessed fats like butter, ghee or virgin olive oil that will make you feel full sooner and will provide important nutrients for your brain and body.

Why do I suggest you make your own food plan? Because it needs to work for you! We all have likes and dislikes and very different lifestyles, so a specific food plan that works for me will not necessarily work for you, even if they are based on the same rules. And if we make our own plan, we are much more likely to commit to it and make it happen.

Once you have done that, make sure that you have the ingredients you need for your food plan for at least the first week. It is also important to stock up with healthy snacks, so that if you do find yourself hungry, these are readily available to you. Equally important is to remove from the house the foods and drinks that you are trying to avoid consuming. This is especially important for any foods that you feel addicted to and for the sugary or starchy snacks that you eat if you get peckish. If possible, encourage others in your household to support you by also doing away with unhealthy foods. If they are unwilling to, ask them to respect your chosen eating plan, and ask if they would refrain from eating or drinking items you wish to avoid, when in your presence.

It can be very lonely making changes to your diet if everyone else around you is carrying on as before. Is there someone within your household or circle of friends who could also do with improving their health? If so, maybe they would join you as you make changes to your diet. Even if they do not have diabetes, the changes I am suggesting will help protect them from diabetes in the future. If there is no one else who is willing or able to make changes with you, is there someone who you can confide in? Someone who can support you as you start your programme of making changes and encourage you to stick with them.

Finally, please speak to your doctor or diabetes nurse about your medication. It is important to review your diabetes or blood pressure medications when embarking on a change to your diet, as some may need to be adjusted, to prevent your blood glucose or blood pressure falling too quickly. If you do take blood pressure medications, then I recommend that you buy a monitor so you can check your blood pressure at home. They are relatively inexpensive and can be bought online or from your local pharmacy. This is covered in more detail in Chapter 13.

Managing food addiction

In Chapter 4, we discussed the fact that many of us develop addictive behaviours towards certain foods. If you think there are some foods that you are addicted to and will have difficulty avoiding, a useful starting point is to list them and call them your 'drug foods' or 'trigger foods'. These are the foods that you feel you can't stop eating. These are the foods that, in addiction theory, are described as the foods where 'one bite is too many and a thousand is never enough'. A very important lesson is captured in that sentence: if you can avoid putting it in your mouth and tasting it, it will not have the chance to trigger you to keep eating. In other words, abstinence, or giving it up completely, is the only solution that works, not cutting down or eating in moderation. That means, for example, that if ice cream is a trigger food, then you need to stop eating it completely. Just like you would not advise an alcoholic to only have one or two whiskies a week, those of us who exhibit addictive symptoms and behaviours associated with certain foods need to learn that we cannot moderate or cut down our intake of these foods. If we want to win back control over what and how much we eat, we need to put ourselves in a position where our brains are not 'hijacked' by these foods, causing us to be controlled by them instead of the other way around.

This might sound terrifying and totally impossible to you. In fact, as far as I know, all food addicts go through this stage of thinking there must be another way. We simply cannot stand the thought of never being able to eat ice cream or milk chocolate again. We are desperate to find another way. But the truth is we have to rewire our brain reward centres and the only way we can do that is by eating foods that will nourish and achieve balance without continuing to trigger massive dopamine rushes.

We must do it in baby steps, one day at a time. Setting a goal for the day, not for the month or the year. Just making sure we stay 'abstinent' for the day today. Tell yourself in the morning, as you get up: Just today, I will not eat my 'drug food'. Then do it again tomorrow… and the next day. Over time it gets easier. The longer you go without, the stronger you will get and the less you will find that you need it. And we can make it easier for ourselves by finding substitute 'treats' – not necessarily foods.

In fact, what we aim to achieve is to eat to live rather than to live to eat. One of our exciting but tough challenges is to get beyond the obsession we have about certain foods… That question in the back of our minds that some people call the 'chatter' about when I am next going to be able to eat those foods.

That isn't the same as saying that food should not be enjoyable or that we should not anticipate and delight in a good long meal together with friends and family – but it needs to be about more than the food and drink, and also a balanced enjoyment of real, natural healthy foods that we can control and that are not controlling us.

For people who are addicted to certain foods, making your own food plan is even more important. In addition to the guidelines in the previous section, if you struggle with trigger foods, then I also suggest:

- Cut out all your drug and trigger foods on day one. If you have a sugar addiction, the trigger foods will be all sweet or sugary foods; they may also include grain-based foods like breads, cereals and pastas, in which case you will need to cut these out too. Remember, aim to do this for just one day at a time. Congratulate yourself and give yourself a non-food treat when you succeed. Tick the days off a calendar as you go. Be proud when you succeed! Don't despair on the days you fail.
- Be careful with everything sweet, including fruits and sweeteners, ideally abstaining, or starting to force a change of tastes as soon as you can – see below.
- Be careful of nuts and seeds, cheese and cream and be aware that these can cause cravings for some people, and take on 'drug food' qualities, even if previously they did not consider them to be 'drug foods'.
- Be brave and tell people you don't eat certain foods and that you are 'intolerant' of them. Anyone who has an allergy has no fear of telling people this. Those of us who are food addicts

will over time hold our heads up and become brave enough to tell people that we are not tolerant of certain types of foods.

- Make as much of your food as possible from scratch and be prepared to experiment with herbs and spices, raw and cooked, soups and salads, etc., favouring savoury over sweet at all times.

Planning ahead is key. That might seem at odds with the advice I have just given about 'taking one day at a time'. But it is not. Planning ahead helps us make sure we have the right foods available, know when and what we intend to eat, and anticipate situations that could be risky for us. And planning is also about more than the food – what activities we want to fill our lives with, so we are excited and occupied with non-eating or non-food-obsessing activities that we enjoy or can learn to enjoy.

Identifying bad habits and trying to replace them with good ones is another important key. Habits sustain themselves, so they are one of the most powerful tools in our toolbox that will help us achieve what we want without huge effort. The effort comes during the process of forcing a change and practising it, but once this forced change starts to become habitual, it gathers momentum and becomes easy. A forced change to drink a glass of water or boil the kettle and make a cup of tea every time you feel 'peckish', instead of going to the biscuit tin, may sound impossible, but it is not. Force it enough times and it becomes a new habit with the benefit that the longer you are 'abstinent' from eating those biscuits, the easier it becomes to avoid them.

Forcing changes of tastes is also a great opportunity for us. Most of us have foods we don't like. Imagine how wonderful it would be if we could get to a point where we don't actually like the foods that caused us problems in the first place.

This takes time and effort and involves being tough with yourself, but it also works. I know of one person who forced herself to eat 85 per cent chocolate with the milk chocolate she used to live on, and for every piece of milk chocolate she ate, she forced herself to eat a piece of dark chocolate with it. Over a few weeks she changed the proportions to eat less and less of the milk chocolate, which meant she became less and less tempted to eat it. As with forcing changes of habits, the resulting 'abstinence' from eating the sweet milk chocolate meant she had fewer cravings. If you drink sugary drinks, try watering them down (using sparkling water if they are carbonated drinks), to slowly wean yourself off the sweetness that you have developed a taste for. Hypnotists like Paul McKenna also provide ideas for how to use your imagination to think of these foods as mixed with hairs from a barbershop (yuck!). One person created the expression 'this is not my food, it's the dog food'… And not many of us would be tempted to eat dog food.

One of the UK's leading experts on food addiction is Heidi Giaever (www.huntsland-nutrition.com) who has kindly allowed me to share her advice on relapses. Heidi says, 'Don't make the mistake of thinking dealing with food addiction is a "quick fix" job that involves a "wash and go" type solution or just "white knuckling it" for a few weeks. While it is important that we celebrate every small success on this tough journey, we mustn't count our chickens too soon or make the mistake of thinking that once we start to feel the cravings are subsiding and we are in more control, that this is it, we've cracked it!'

Heidi emphasizes the importance of relapse prevention planning and says it is very important to map risky situations and make sure we anticipate the danger zones that might throw us off balance and trigger a relapse. She encourages people to make a Relapse

Prevention Plan. If you struggle with any degree of food addiction, I really recommend spending some time preparing your own plan. The plan should identify every imaginable situation in which you could find yourself, when you might be tempted, let your guard down or be at risk of being persuaded that 'one won't hurt', etc. The plan should also include a set of pre-prepared 'I WILL' statements that are intended to snap into action when the risky situations arise. In constructing your plan, consider the following questions and write your answers for each one. If possible, find a close friend who wants to help you and ask them what they would do if they were faced with your challenges. Add to this list whenever you learn new insights about yourself and when listening to the experiences or suggestions you like from others:

1. When might a relapse happen?

2. What circumstances or triggers are likely to be present?

3. Is anyone else likely to be involved?

4. Will there be any warning signs before it happens?

5. What safety nets can you prepare for yourself (people, decisions, other)?

As an example, you might feel that a relapse could happen when you are feeling sad or sorry for yourself. You might be aware that you get such feelings if you see your weight creeping up and you feel despondent. Maybe your partner will be involved and notice that you are feeling bad. They might even take pity and suggest you have a treat to perk yourself up. Warning signs could be that you know when you get 'low' because you feel tired and have no energy. Safety nets could include having a bag of your favourite nuts readily available to keep you from the cakes or chocolates; or preparing a non-food-related treat to congratulate yourself for staying on track.

Then have a think about the rules you will set yourself to help you avoid or manage a relapse. These are your simple rules that you decide upon in advance, knowing that there is a reasonable chance you will face situations where you fall back into behaviours that you have decided to change. What will you do if you face such situations? These rules can be anything – from going out for a walk, having a long soak in the bath, listening to music. It doesn't matter what they are, as long as they are realistic and that you like them. You can rewrite these rules any time, as you learn what works and what doesn't.

1. I will…

2. I will…

3. I will…

Then, write down two or three encouraging reminders or treats that you should use to make sure you do not let one small relapse get you down. These are your decisions, based on knowing yourself and what motivates and inspires you to get around any negative or self-destructive thinking.

1. I will encourage myself to…

2. I will remind myself that…

3. I will treat myself by…

It is important to make this a process that you learn from each time you practise it. Sometimes we think we have a plan that will work in certain situations, then when it comes to it, it fails completely for some reason. We must learn from this, think about what would work better and change the plan accordingly.

If you are someone who recognizes the value of having someone to confide in when times are tough, or even a buddy who can take over and be strong for you when you feel weak and are about to succumb, then find that person and help them understand the role you need them to play for you. This is one of the fundamental pillars of organizations such as Alcoholics Anonymous and Overeaters Anonymous. They recommend you find a sponsor who you can call on to offer support within their organization.

Finally, one of the most powerful things we can do for ourselvesin the process of trying to take control of the foods that control us, is to spend time thinking about what it is we truly want in life. Heidi's motto in life is 'Happy are those who dream dreams and are willing to pay the price to make them come true.' These words were on a poster given to her as a young child and they stuck with her and hugely influenced her work. They are very relevant, as that is what fighting and conquering food addiction is all about: finding happiness in the process of dreaming the dream of true freedom from these foods and understanding how and what to do, to make this dream come true. Dr Jen Unwin – in her book on conquering food addiction, *Fork in the Road* – talks about the power of hope, and I see this very much as powering ourselves with positive psychology, knowing all the things we have managed to accomplish in the past, from passing an exam to being thanked by someone who appreciates what we do for them. Reminding ourselves of our achievements, however small they may seem to us; recognizing them as real strengths and capacities and building on these to become stronger than the addictive powers of trigger foods and to be able to push them away, knowing they harm us and have no place in our future of true happiness and freedom.

When I last looked, there were more than 260 million google hits against the words 'food addiction', which shows how immensely important this subject is and how those who recognize themselves as food addicts are not alone in this world. There are also growing numbers of organizations and educated counsellors who can help with structure and support. Many individuals work internationally and can be reached via the Food Addiction Institute and Bitten's Addiction.[38]

But even without the help of a trained counsellor, you can employ a few simple tricks to get yourself on the right road to recovery, following the guidance above and remembering a few basic facts about food addiction:

- Moderation therapy will seldom, if ever, work. Abstinence from 'drug' and 'trigger' foods is the best start and end point.

- Relapses will happen in the early days, so make this your best learning experience and use it to make your Relapse Prevention Plan more robust and practically suited to you and your life than it was previously.

- Don't think you can solve this overnight. Just as with insulin resistance and prediabetes or type 2 diabetes, the disease of food addiction has probably been deeply established over decades, possibly since childhood. It requires effort and perseverance to undo the damage.

Undoing the damage is very possible and there are increasing amounts of resources and publications available to help. If you have read this, you will already have some of the tools developing in your mind for how to start taking the small steps needed in the right direction. Start by taking one day at a time and do not let yourself be overpowered by the fear or anger you may feel at the thought of abstinence from your favourite foods. Forget about the long term for now. Just make the decision TODAY that you will not eat your drug or trigger foods – just for today! Then make the same decision tomorrow…

Staying on track

Once you have started to make changes, you will hopefully begin to see some results to reward you for your effort. It is likely that you will soon see that your blood glucose levels will start coming down and your clothes will feel a little looser. Indeed, one of the most common complaints I hear is people saying they have to buy new trousers as their old ones will no longer stay up! As you experience these positive benefits, take some time to reflect on your progress, to tell yourself what a good job you have done and to encourage yourself to continue the good work.

For some people, reducing sugars and starches can be quite a shock to the system and might cause some side effects. These are usually only temporary, and they disappear as your system gets used to its 'new normal'. However, they may be disconcerting and so it is important that you are aware of them, and what you can do about them, to avoid them getting you down and losing faith in your new way of eating.

Perhaps the most common symptom is a feeling of fatigue. This can last for one to two weeks, but it will pass. Make sure you get a good night's sleep (see Chapter 14) and try not to over-exert yourself while your body is adapting to your new diet. It can be associated with headaches and sometimes light-headedness. Reducing carbohydrates can lead to an increase in urine production, causing mild dehydration and a reduction in blood pressure. Ensure that you drink plenty of water each day. You may also benefit from adding some extra salt to your meals each day (maybe ½ a teaspoon on each of two meals).

Some people experience muscle cramps, because of changes to the levels of chemicals, such as sodium, potassium and magnesium, in the muscle cells. These too are usually helped by adding extra salt. If they persist, then taking a magnesium supplement, such as magnesium citrate or glycinate, for a couple of weeks usually does the trick. Finally, some people experience constipation. This is likely because of mild dehydration and usually resolves within a couple of weeks. It can be improved by drinking plenty of water and by taking magnesium supplements. You can also use a laxative for a while if required.

I would reiterate that these symptoms are a natural reaction to your body adjusting to your new diet. If you are aware that they might occur, you can drink plenty of water and, if necessary, increase your salt intake, and you should find they pass without causing undue anxiety or making you lose momentum with the changes you are making.

When I was working in Bermuda, many patients asked me if they could have a cheat day; others had already decided that, for example, Saturday was their 'cheat day'. It was not a concept I had heard of before. I think it comes from people who have been on various restrictive diets and allowed themselves a cheat day so that they could indulge in their favourite foods once in a while. The trouble with a cheat day every week is that it risks undoing all the good that you have done in the previous six days. And if you indulge in your trigger foods on cheat days, then you will not succeed in breaking their hold on you. Therefore, and at risk of seeming harsh, my answer is NO cheat days. If you want to turn your health around, the goal must be to make permanent changes to your lifestyle. For the changes to be permanent, you must be able to enjoy your new way of eating, without craving the foods that helped cause your ill health in the first place. So, instead of a food-related cheat day, how about a non-food treat day once a week, when you will treat yourself for staying on track. It could be a walk in the park, having coffee with a friend or going to the cinema. Some weeks you might wish to work out how much you have saved by not buying takeaways or cakes and spend the money on a small gift – just for you.

Getting back on track

The changes you need to make to reverse type 2 diabetes or prediabetes need to be long term. Day in, day out; week in, week out; and, of course, year in, year out. We have already discussed how addiction to 'trigger' foods requires great willpower and plans put in place to maximize the chances of success and minimize the risk of sliding back into old habits. Some people, whose affiliation with sugary or starchy foods might not be as strong as an addiction, can find it relatively easy to change their eating habits, once they understand the benefits. Indeed, while I and many others run intensive courses to help people switch to and stay on a low-carb diet, these are not always necessary. Many people achieved success after reading my book *Reverse Your Diabetes*. Still others achieved success after one consultation with me. A few stand out. One was a man, well into his eighties, with whom I had a telephone consultation during the 2020 coronavirus lockdown. His HbA1c was very high and he did not want to take additional medications. During the 15-minute consultation, I was able to suggest some simple changes he could make in order to reduce his carbohydrate intake and thus avoid the need for more medications. He made those changes and, as a result, after just three months, his HbA1c had reduced by 33 mmol/mol, or 3 per cent. Not only does this show that some people, given the correct information, can make changes quite easily, it also shows that you are never too old to make lifestyle changes.

For others, though, it can be a bit more complex. Even if we do not feel addicted to certain foods, many of us find change – any change – very difficult. Take one example. For many years, we have been led to believe that porridge is healthy. As a cereal, it probably is the least bad one there is, but if you have diabetes, then it is likely to cause a rise in blood glucose level. That's why I suggest switching away from all forms of cereal, and to a breakfast based on protein and healthy fat, such as eggs or plain Greek yoghurt. I can recall a number of people who made this switch quite successfully, but three months later they were back on porridge. It wasn't that they didn't like their new breakfast, it was because their brains had been wired for decades to believe that porridge was their breakfast, and perhaps without consciously deciding to, they reverted to their decades-old habit. It really is an example of 'old habits die hard'.

Still others deviate from their low-carbohydrate eating pattern because something else comes along that just changes everything. I have had patients who have been doing really well who then experienced major 'life events' – including the death of a spouse, a diagnosis of cancer, and loss of employment or housing. I hardly need to explain how any one of these can be such a shock to the system that it will materially impact on a person's ability to stay on track with their new way of eating. While it might be possible to plan for a relapse for situations where you might be tempted in normal daily life – for example, if you are planning to attend a birthday celebration – I am not sure that any of us can adequately plan for the impact of a major life event. We all live with the possibility that something awful might happen to ourselves or to a loved one – unfortunately, 'that's life', or as someone once put it to me, 'shit happens'. So rather than trying to plan ahead, the key when this happens is to accept that life has thrown a spanner in the works, manage the immediate impact on your diabetes and when the time is right, plan how you can get back on track. So, what does this mean in practice?

First of all, I encourage everyone in this situation to focus on everything they have achieved up until that point. All the weight they have lost, the reduction in their blood glucose levels, the reductions in their medications, the improvement in how they feel. Sometimes it is helpful to list them all and write them down. Then acknowledge that it is entirely natural to be thrown off course by what has happened. Do not beat yourself up about it. However, if, as a result of what has happened to you and your eating patterns or stress levels, your glucose levels have shot up, please seek advice about managing them – if necessary, with medications, at least in the short term. Once life begins to return to normal, you may well be able to come off them again.

In my experience, for most people in this situation, life does return to something more normal, and in each of the cases I mentioned earlier, that person was able to get back on track with their eating pattern. However, it will likely take some time, and this is exactly the moment to seek the help of a close friend or health professional who can provide you with emotional support as you work through the life event, and then begin to plan how to get back on track. In Chapter 1, I touched on the importance of setting your goal in a way that gives you hope for a brighter future. If life has thrown a spanner in the works, it may be difficult to regain that sense of hope in the same way. However, if you find yourself in that situation, I suggest you reread Chapter 1, and start again by setting yourself a new goal, based on your changed situation and your new hopes for a healthier future.

This happened to Steve, who shared his story at the end of Chapter 3. Having lost weight and reversed his diabetes and his retinopathy, his world changed. In 2018, his wife died after a short illness caused by a cancer that had been diagnosed some years before. He says, 'In my grief, I found it difficult to maintain the diet changes and I began to put weight back on. I just let myself go and it felt as though I no longer had any willpower. The diabetic eye disease came back in one eye, and I did need some injections. Thankfully, it has now cleared up. I now have the support of a close friend who is helping me get back onto the diet and to stay on track.'

Finally, whether you are just starting out, or have been on a journey of change for some time, there is plenty of support available on various diabetes forums on the internet. There is almost always someone who has been through a similar experience to yours, and who can offer advice based on their own experiences.

Richard attended a course run by Heidi Giaever, who contributed significantly to this chapter. Read how her guidance helped him to overcome an addictive relationship with food and to reverse his type 2 diabetes.

RICHARD'S STORY

Years of weight and health problems meant I was 134 kg (295 pounds) at retirement. Loss of mobility contributed; a larger part was unhealthy diet. Weight-loss attempts were only temporarily successful. Keeping weight off was impossible – I was in a worsening cycle. Overeating, large portions and comfort eating for high stress were the problems. Binge eating of sugary foods – buying a pack of four meant eating them all at once – and convenience foods became habitual. I wanted to be slimmer, but not enough to change my habits.

My nurse suggested the standard NHS recommenda-tions: a low-fat, high-carb diet, plenty of fruit/veg and 'more exercise'. Extremely difficult with fibromyalgia and fatigue. I moved from prediabetic to type 2 diabetes in 2018, with blood pressure at 145/95. Metformin was prescribed. The diagnosis was not a shock, and I largely ignored it.

Then in December 2020 my GP invited me to a diabetes programme. I weighed 122 kg (269 pounds), my HbA1c was 48 (6.5 per cent) and waistline 114 cm (45 inches). I learnt that the NHS guideline was wrong for 'diabetic me' on every level! I was consuming a lot of fruit as a 'healthy' substitute for sugar/carbs, chocolate and biscuits, but only making my insulin resistance worse. I identified that my trigger foods were pastries and sweet biscuits which I consumed too much and too often. I needed to exclude these completely because I couldn't trust myself not to overeat them if they were in the house. This was difficult at first but has become easier. Retraining my brain seems to have been successful, but I still won't have them in my home. The other food I really miss is fruit which I ate for its supposed health benefits without realizing the sugar load. I miss bananas, nectarines and grapes the most. I have eaten two bananas in the last six months, so far without triggering a craving/habit again.

Changing shopping lists and diet was vital to regaining health. Being given clear science-based explanations was essential. In eight weeks, I lost 9.5 kg (21 pounds) and my waistline was 112 cm (44 inches). My HbA1c at 48.6 (6.6 per cent) was disappointingly static, but I was motivated to expect improvement. Indeed, six months later my weight was down to 104 kg (229 pounds), waist 109 cm (43 inches) and HbA1c 41 (5.9 per cent). Seven pairs of trousers were now too big! My metformin prescription was discontinued and my type 2 is now in remission!

My introduction to the concept of food addiction opened my mind to social engineering in the food industry. No wonder ultra-processed junk tastes good. Analysing my habits, risk factors and upbringing (I hate wasting food... I like to try new things... I had no food discipline) was illuminating and helped me improve my eating habits. I have a 'dream timeline' mind map that charts my progress. In my plan to avoid relapse, I have made choices about where to shop and which aisles to avoid; and where foods and beverages are kept thus reducing 'casual' snacking. I now feel full after eating, so feel less compulsion to snack. My tastes are already changing and I no longer need the sugar rush or short-lived satisfaction of tempting carbs. I am confident of reaching my target and staying in remission. A low-carb, high-fat diet with fresh real ingredients in place of processed foods has seen me lose 18 kg (40 pounds) in six months, and I intend to lose another 6 kg (13 pounds) in the next six months. The support group is valuable for encouragement and motivation.

Addictive behaviour develops in subtle ways. My body had craved toxic sugar, forcing me into insulin resistance. Following the programme means I no longer crave sugary foods. I have adapted to minimum carbs and enjoy cooking with fresh ingredients. Being inventive with real food recipes is reprogramming my mind and body. I am reclaiming my independence and rewiring my brain.

An additional benefit is improved general health. I am still physically restricted, subject to chronic pain and fatigue, but I can walk further, garden (slowly) and enjoy my hobby of outdoor photography. For the first time, I am confident that weight loss and better health are achievable and worth the effort and the deliberate change of tastes and habits. I can be 80 kg (176 pounds) and fitter in three years. I CAN do it!

CHAPTER 13

The role of medication

If you have prediabetes, it is unlikely that you will have been prescribed diabetes medication, as diet changes are usually sufficient to reverse the condition. Some people with prediabetes are treated with metformin (described below) which can be continued while you make diet changes. Once you have reversed the condition, it can usually be stopped.

If you are on medication for blood pressure, then it is important for this to be reviewed by your doctor as you start to make dietary changes, as your medication may need to be reduced or stopped. I always recommend that people on such medication have their own monitor, so they can check their blood pressure themselves (see Chapter 16).

Otherwise, if you have prediabetes or type 2 diabetes and you are not on any diabetes medications, this chapter will not be relevant to you, and you can move on to Chapter 14 about your mental health.

Medications for type 2 diabetes

Over the past 20 years a number of new medications have been developed to treat type 2 diabetes; as a result, there are now plenty of options, and they work in various ways. This is very different from the situation when I first started working in diabetes, when there were essentially three possibilities: metformin, a group of drugs called sulfonylureas (which make the pancreas produce extra insulin) and insulin itself. Given our current understanding, that the main problem in type 2 diabetes is that there is too much insulin, it really does not make sense to use treatments that increase insulin still further as this will make it almost impossible for a person using these treatments to reverse their diabetes. Sulfonylureas and insulin are therefore used much less nowadays.

The first of the original trio – metformin – is still very much in use, however. In fact, although it is one of the oldest diabetes treatments available (it was first used in the 1950s), in almost every treatment guideline from around the world, it is recommended as the first drug to be prescribed for people with type 2 diabetes. Unlike sulfonylureas, metformin does not increase the amount of insulin the pancreas produces, rather it helps the body use its own insulin more effectively, thus reducing insulin resistance. This means the pancreas does not need to produce so much insulin in order to control blood glucose levels, and less insulin makes it easier to lose weight.

Two other types of drug commonly in use today, dipeptidyl peptidase 4 (DPP4) inhibitors and glucagon-like peptide-1 (GLP1) analogues, also work by reducing insulin resistance. Pioglitazone is another drug that reduces insulin resistance, but as it causes weight gain and other side effects, it is used less often now. The newest diabetes drugs are known as sodium glucose transporter 2 (SGLT2) inhibitors. They work by making the kidneys remove additional glucose from the bloodstream, so that it is excreted in the urine. They therefore reduce blood glucose levels directly, which in turn will reduce the amount of insulin that needs to be produced, and therefore they also help with weight loss. Acarbose, which is rarely used nowadays as it can cause unpleasant gut side effects, reduces glucose levels by stopping it from being absorbed from the gut into the bloodstream.

Because of their impact on reducing the level of insulin in the blood, metformin, DPP4 inhibitors, GLP1 analogues and SGLT2 inhibitors can all help reverse the diabetes disease process. Table 12 lists all the drugs currently used to treat type 2 diabetes in the UK (in 2021). Note that all have side effects. In many people these are relatively mild, such as nausea or abdominal bloating. Some drugs, in certain situations, can have quite serious side effects. The SGLT2 inhibitors, for example, are effective in improving glucose levels and helping people lose weight, and they are also good for the heart and kidneys. However, they can be associated with increased risk of foot amputation, and in people on a low-carbohydrate diet, they can be associated with a serious metabolic condition known as diabetic ketoacidosis. It is therefore essential that everyone who takes medications is aware of the potential side effects, so they can make an informed decision about whether that medicine is right for them. Metformin and SGLT2 inhibitors cannot be used in people with significantly reduced kidney function, or when they become acutely unwell. This will be discussed in more detail in Chapter 15.

ble 12: Medications for type 2 diabetes

rug names	Brand name	How it is given	Side effects
iguanide			
1etformin	Glucophage	Tablet 1–2x daily	*Common:* diarrhoea, bloating
PP4 inhibitors			
ogliptin	Nesina	Tablet 1x daily	*Rare:* pancreatitis
nagliptin	Trajenta		
axagliptin	Onglyza		
tagliptin	Januvia		
Idagliptin	Galvus		
LP1 analogues			
xenatide	Byetta Bydureon	Injection 2x daily Injection 1x weekly	*Common:* reduced appetite, nausea, vomiting
raglutide	Victoza	Injection 1x daily	*Rare:* pancreatitis
xisenatide	Lyxumia	Injection 1x daily	
ulaglutide	Trulicity	Injection 1x weekly	
maglutide	Ozempic	Injection 1x weekly	
	Rybelsus	Tablet 1x daily	
iLT2 inhibitors			
anagliflozin	Invokana	Tablet 1x daily	*Common:* urinary infections, thrush
apagliflozin	Forxiga		*Rare:* ketoacidosis, amputation, gangrene
npagliflozin	Jardiance		
pha glucosidase inhibitor			
arbose	Glucobay	Tablet 3x daily	*Common:* flatulence
iazolidinedione			
oglitazone	Actos	Tablet 1x daily	*Common:* weight gain *Rare:* fractures, bladder cancer
eglitinides			
paglinide	Prandin	Tablet 3x daily	*Common:* low blood glucose, weight gain *Rare:* abdominal pain, diarrhoea
Ifonylureas			
benclamide	Daonil	Tablet 1x daily	*Common:* low blood glucose, weight gain
mepiride	Amaryl	Tablet 1x daily	*Rare:* abdominal pain, diarrhoea
clazide	Diamicron	Tablet 1–2x daily	
pizide	Glucotrol	Tablet 1–2x daily	
butamide	Orinase	Tablet 2–3x daily	
ulins			
ious types		Injection 1–4x daily	*Common:* low blood glucose, weight gain

Deprescribing medications when reversing type 2 diabetes

If you choose to reverse your diabetes by going onto a very low-calorie diet, then it is usually recommended that you stop all your diabetes medications when you start the low-calorie phase. This should be done under medical supervision, as other medications, such as for blood pressure, may also need to be reduced. This approach also requires a significant reduction in dose for people on insulin injections.

If you are using a low-carbohydrate diet as recommended in this book, then it is important to ensure that, as you make changes to your diet, your blood glucose levels do not fall too low. That may mean that you will need to reduce some of your medications.

The top priority is to reduce medications that increase insulin in the blood circulation or cause weight gain, as these will get in the way of your attempt to reverse the diabetes disease process. That means reducing the dose of pioglitazone and any insulin, sulfonylurea or meglitinide that you are taking. My general advice is to halve the dose as you start to reduce your carbohydrate intake. These changes should be done in conjunction with your doctor or diabetes nurse, especially if you are on more than one type of diabetes medication. As your glucose levels come down, you will hopefully be able to stop some or all of these medications altogether.

If you are on one or more of the other medications in Table 12, then these can all be continued as you begin to reduce your carbohydrate intake. If you reduce your carbohydrate intake below 75 g per day, then it is recommended to stop SGLT2 inhibitors, because of the increased risk of diabetic ketoacidosis associated with a low-carbohydrate diet. Therefore, if you plan quickly to embark on a very low-carbohydrate diet, then any SGLT2 inhibitor that you take should be stopped before you start to reduce your carbohydrates. Other medications can then be reduced or stopped, as your blood glucose levels fall. I generally suggest making a change if your fasting blood glucose is generally around 7 mmol/l (125 mg/dl) or less. A suggested order to do this would be to stop acarbose (if taking it), then a DPP4 inhibitor. Staying on a GLP1 analogue can be effective, particularly if you have a lot of weight to lose, as it helps to suppress appetite. However, that too can be stopped once you are well on your way to achieving your weight goal and/or once your HbA1c is below 48 mmol/mol (6.5 per cent). The final drug to stop is metformin. Remember, if you can come off all your diabetes medications and maintain your HbA1c below 48 mmol/mol or 6.5 per cent, for at least three months, then by definition your diabetes is in remission. Remember also, that if you revert to your previous eating pattern, your glucose levels will go up again, and you may need to restart medication. Just as type 2 diabetes is a reversible condition, remission is also reversible.

Table 13 (page 237) shows the medication changes that should be considered when starting a low-carbohydrate diet. This is adapted from a paper that I co-authored, published in 2019.[39] I reiterate that it is essential to discuss your medications with your GP or diabetes nurse, as each person may have individual requirements that need to be taken into account.

Blood pressure medications

Many people with prediabetes and type 2 diabetes need to take medications for high blood pressure. This is because the high insulin levels that occur in people with type 2 diabetes and prediabetes cause the body to retain more sodium (salt) in the blood. The high salt level in turn means the body retains more water in the circulation and that increases blood pressure. When you eat less carbohydrate, the insulin levels fall. This in turn means the salt levels fall, less water is in the circulation and blood pressure reduces. If you are on blood pressure medications, it is therefore very important to monitor your blood pressure using an automatic machine, and if necessary, reduce your blood pressure medications as your blood pressure falls. Please seek the advice of your doctor or nurse about this.

Other medications

Warfarin is an anticoagulant that reduces the ability of the blood to clot. It is usually prescribed to people who have had a blood clot in the past. It has largely been replaced by more modern drugs, but if you do take warfarin, it is important to be aware that, if you increase your intake of green vegetables that contain vitamin K (such as kale, spinach, sprouts and broccoli), it can reduce the effect of warfarin and the dose may need to be increased.

As you lose weight and your blood glucose control improves, then you may find that other health problems apart from high blood pressure also begin to improve. I have known people come off medications for joint pains, acid reflux, gout and erectile dysfunction as a result of adopting a low-carbohydrate diet. This is great for the individuals concerned, as well as for the health service that no longer has to pay for so many medications. It also shows just how many health problems arise from being overweight or metabolically unhealthy.

Table 13: A guide to deprescribing medications

Priority to reduce or stop	Class of drug	Changes when starting a low-carbohydrate diet
1	Insulins (various types)	Generally, halve the dose when starting a low-carbohydrate diet. Doses can then be reduced as glucose levels fall below 7 mmol/l (125 mg/dl). If glucose levels then rise, revert to the previous dose, and seek professional advice.
1–3	SGLT2 inhibitors (e.g. canagliflozin)	Must be stopped if total carbohydrate intake is less than 75 g per day. Otherwise, it can be reduced and eventually stopped if fasting glucose levels fall below 7 mmol/l (125 mg/dl).
2	Sulfonylureas (e.g. gliclazide)	Halve the dose when starting a low-carbohydrate diet. Stop if fasting glucose levels fall below 7 mmol/l (125 mg/dl).
2	Meglitinides (repaglinide)	Halve the dose when starting a low-carbohydrate diet. Stop if fasting glucose levels fall below 7 mmol/l (125 mg/dl).
3	Thiazolidinedione (pioglitazone)	Halve the dose when starting a low-carbohydrate diet. Stop if fasting glucose levels fall below 7 mmol/l (125 mg/dl).
4	Alpha glucosidase inhibitor (acarbose)	No change initially. Stop if fasting glucose levels fall below 7 mmol/l (125 mg/dl).
5	DPP4 inhibitors (e.g. sitagliptin)	No change initially. Can be stopped if fasting glucose levels fall below 7 mmol/l (125 mg/dl).
6	GLP1 analogues (e.g. liraglutide)	No change initially. Can be reduced and eventually stopped if fasting glucose levels fall below 7 mmol/l (125 mg/dl). Can be continued to help weight loss.
7	Biguanide (metformin)	No change. Can be stopped if HbA1c is below 48 mmol/mol (6.5 per cent).
According to blood pressure	Blood pressure medications (various types)	Generally, reduce dose if systolic blood pressure is consistently less than 120.

VIVIAN'S STORY

I am 76 years old and have had type 2 diabetes for about 20 years. When I was first diagnosed, I was told that eventually I would have to go on to insulin. 'Everyone does.' Sure enough, after several years of trying metformin and other drugs, that made me put on weight alarmingly, I was on insulin. At first it scared me and I hated doing it but because my sugar levels were reduced I became accustomed to it and accepted it. This was my way of life now.

In December 2020, I was asked if I would like to attend a new programme to help people get off their diabetic medication and that I would be on 20 g of carbohydrates a day. I immediately got my scales out and started checking the amount of carbs in everything that I ate. I kept a very strict food diary. I have always cooked and I now do batch cooking to freeze portions that are weighed and labelled with carbs per portion. This way I know exactly what I am consuming.

I started this course 4 February 2021, my GOLDEN DAY, and haven't looked back. When I started I was on 44 units of insulin a day. A few weeks before, the nurse told me to cut my insulin to 30 units a day. A bit scary, but I did it and nothing happened. On 16 February, she said to drop it to 15 units, and on 22 February she said STOP taking insulin! That was a really scary thing to do! NO INSULIN! I was very worried initially, but my sugar levels were mostly between 5 and 6. I could not believe it. Then on 26 February she suggested I stop taking dapagliflozin. My sugar levels are mostly between 7 and 8 and very stable, not all over the place as they used to be. I am still on metformin but am hoping that eventually I will reach a level where I can stop that too.

So far, I have lost 16 kg (35 pounds). I was not interested in weight loss, I just wanted to reduce my medication, but it has been a pleasant side effect. My blood pressure has come down to normal, so I think I might be able to come off that medication as well. This really is the best thing I have ever done for my health and I only wish I had known about it years ago.

There are times when I really fancy something sweet. To stop myself picking, I eat three times a day, and am never hungry. I know that my danger time is about 4 pm, so I put the kettle on and make myself a cup of Bovril. That stops me wanting sweet things. I find a hot drink fills me up too.

I will keep eating this way forever. Any temptations and I think how life was just a few months ago, and how much better I feel now. I know I will never go back to my old eating habits.

CHAPTER 14

Looking after your mental health

We all feel low from time to time – and often for good reason. We are, after all, complicated beings with complex emotions. It is a normal part of being human. However, you can't have helped noticing that mental health problems are on the increase. Between 2007 and 2014, the prevalence of depression in the UK increased by over 40 per cent and of anxiety by over 30 per cent. In 2016, the UK national health service spent over £64 million on antidepressants, nearly £4 million more than the previous year. The issues surrounding mental health are very multifaceted, and within those numbers are many people with serious mental health problems that require specialist treatment. However, increasingly, we are aware that our lifestyle can affect our mental health and vice versa, and this gives us some important clues about lifestyle changes we can make to improve our mental health, as well as our physical health.

There is now plenty of evidence that there is a link between poor mental health and obesity, prediabetes and type 2 diabetes. It is recognized that people who are overweight are often unhappy about themselves and may experience feelings of shame or guilt. This is not helped by the perception of many that such problems are self-inflicted. But there is also evidence that insulin resistance itself can affect the chemical balance in the brain and increase the likelihood of symptoms of depression.[40] Remember that insulin resistance is found in many people who are overweight, and in almost everyone with either prediabetes or type 2 diabetes.

In some cases, severe obesity results from comfort eating as a coping strategy to help deal with past traumatic events. However, perhaps much more common is the use of sweet foods as a pick-me-up if we are feeling a bit down or just want to cheer ourselves up. As we discussed in Chapter 12, sugar has a direct effect on the brain and causes a feeling of wellbeing. On brain scans, it lights up the same parts of the brain as some drugs do. Some people call it a sugar rush. Others describe getting sugar cravings, as the effect wears off, leading them to eat yet more – a sort of withdrawal reaction that leads some people to consider that they have an addiction, either to sugar or sometimes also to other carbohydrate-containing foods. A vicious cycle then sets in motion, where a person with insulin resistance is more liable to feeling depressed. They may then resort to eating sugar-containing foods to improve their mood (which it does in the very short term). However, this also worsens the insulin resistance, which can lead to even lower mood, more sugar intake and so on. And as we know, as well as affecting mood, insulin resistance also increases body weight, blood glucose levels and the risk of prediabetes and then type 2 diabetes.

Food and mental health

There are also links between eating processed foods and having poor mental health. A diet that is low in nutrition and high in processed foods has been associated with an increased risk of depression and mild cognitive impairment.[41] The brain is 60 per cent fat and contains a high concentration of omega-3 fatty acids. Many 'Western' diets are high in omega-6 fatty acids and lower in omega-3 fatty acids and have been associated with an increased risk of depressive disorders. Activation of the immune system to increase inflammation in the body is associated with a greater risk of depression. Guess what – the foods most associated with inflammation include sugar and refined carbohydrates. Margarine (often high in omega-6 fatty acids), red meat and diet soft drinks are also associated with increased inflammation in the body. The foods that were least associated with inflammation included wine, coffee, olive oil and vegetables.

Therefore, not only do sugar and other processed foods increase the risk of prediabetes and type 2 diabetes, they also increase the risk of depression. There is clear evidence of a two-way link between unhealthy diet and poor mental health. Poor mental health can lead to unhealthy eating – but also an unhealthy diet can contribute to poor mental health. We also know that poor mental health can be associated with other unhealthy behaviours, such as being physically inactive. In some people, poor mental health can lead to excessive drinking of alcohol, or even the use of illicit drugs. And as with unhealthy eating, even in people who would not consider themselves addicts, overconsumption of any of these things means their addictive effects can lead to a vicious cycle, which results in worsening symptoms and increasing substance abuse.

That all sounds very depressing, doesn't it? However, the good news is that, just as an improving diet has been shown to reverse the changes that lead to type 2 diabetes, it has also been shown to improve mental health. A healthy diet of fresh, unprocessed foods, avoiding sugars and refined carbohydrates, will help reduce insulin resistance and inflammation, improving both physical and mental health.

I want to make it clear that I am not suggesting that all mental health problems can be solved by eating a certain diet. Nor am I suggesting that people shouldn't take antidepressant or other medication. Very often, by definition, people who are depressed have very poor levels of self-worth. In that situation, motivation to make lifestyle changes just isn't there and sometimes a limited course of antidepressant medication can be helpful in treating the symptoms and improving a person's feelings about themselves. That can give them the motivation to make some small steps towards a healthier lifestyle.

What other aspects of a healthier lifestyle can improve mental health? Probably the quickest win is to go out for a walk. Just going out for a short walk can make us feel better, more alert and, unless you got drenched in the rain, also happier. There is evidence of how being in nature improves health – including mood, as it can have a very calming effect on the brain. More intensive exercise such as running, cycling, swimming or working out in a gym increases the production of endorphins – nature's own opium, and can also have a positive effect on mood.

Reducing stress

Many of us feel as though we are in a constant state of stress. In fact, we might not even feel overtly stressed but the way we live nowadays can lead to a constant state of low-level stress that is harmful to our health. Thirty years ago, for most people, work started and finished when they arrived and left the workplace. Period. Today, with the ubiquitous use of email and ability to send and receive messages, on our mobile phones, we risk being always available. We also risk taking our work home with us, and even to bed with us. The trouble is, for most of us, email has snuck up on us and I guess few of us have ever been trained in how to manage it.

To mobile phones and email, we can add the impact of computer games, 24/7 TV, Netflix box sets, and internet shopping and banking, which all have the potential to raise stress levels or disturb our sleep or both. And none of these things existed 30 years ago!

In many respects, these advances have been beneficial in all sorts of ways. We no longer have to wonder where anyone is, as almost everyone, the world over, now has a personal tracking device, also known as a mobile phone. Yet over these 30 years, as well as seeing increasing rates of obesity and type 2 diabetes, we have also seen increases in a whole host of conditions, including depression, mood disturbances and chronic fatigue. Is modern living that bad for us?

In a word – yes. In previous generations, our lifestyle was dictated by geography and daylight. Without the means to move quickly around, people stayed in relatively close-knit communities and lived and worked close to where they grew up. The world was largely rural and work was necessarily within walking distance. Once it got dark, it was time to switch off the brain and go to sleep – or to stay up in rather dim candlelight. Life wasn't always easy, but it was much closer to the sort of living for which our bodies evolved.

Many of the body's processes are controlled by hormones, which vary according to what is called a circadian rhythm. This means that the hormone levels in the bloodstream change across a 24-hour period. One of the key hormones is cortisol, the body's natural steroid. Its levels rise during the early morning, to ensure that we are wide awake and alert at the start of the day and to prepare us for the day ahead. Then, as the day progresses, cortisol levels naturally decline to reach their lowest levels late at night, to enable the body to sleep.

Cortisol is the body's main stress hormone and is increased whenever we are under any kind of stress. The actions of cortisol are to increase our blood glucose levels and to ratchet up the immune system as part of what is called the fight or flight response, to enable us to fight or run away from an enemy, and to help the body heal following any physical injury. These are all good things if we are in serious trouble, such as being attacked by a wild animal. In that situation, the cortisol level increases to help us survive the attack, then returns down to normal levels.

The trouble is our body's hormones cannot readily distinguish between that type of emergency and the multitude of stresses that impact upon our modern lives. As a result, any emotional, physical or mental stress can cause cortisol levels to spike. It could be as a result of a serious illness, job or money worries, or living in an unhappy relationship. It could also be because of rushing around doing one job after another, getting stuck in traffic or being unfriended on Facebook. The net effect is that all too often we can be in a state of constantly high cortisol levels, meaning our immune system is continually primed and energy stores mobilized to cause blood glucose levels to rise. As we learnt earlier in this chapter, these twin effects of inflammation and insulin resistance are harmful to our mental health, as well as our physical health. By now, you can also see that it stands to reason that, if your cortisol levels are constantly raised, it will make it very difficult to reverse the diabetes disease process. Indeed, many people find that if they are in a stressful situation, their blood glucose levels can go very high indeed – even if they are following a healthy diet. Effectively managing stress is therefore essential, not just for your mental wellbeing, but also for achieving normal glucose levels.

Just as we must learn how to undo the harmful effect of the

unhealthy food that surrounds us, so too – if we really want to maximize our health – must we learn how to undo the harmful effects of our always-on lifestyles. So how can we do that? There are a number of things that will help, some may apply more than others to different people. One that I think is universally relevant is to take breaks during the day. For much of my working life in a busy hospital, I would work for up to ten hours without stopping. I would grab a coffee during the clinic and take it back to my consultation room and I would munch on a sandwich while checking emails at lunchtime. Very often I would spend the entire day in one room. It became normal and I would get home exhausted and not very nice to be with. Now the irony is that the hospital was on a very pleasant green field site, with a large duck pond in the middle. On occasions when I was very stressed, I would go out and walk around the pond, and I recognized it had a calming effect. Now I realize it would have been much better if I had built that into my daily routine.

In 2013, I moved to Belgium and worked in an office environment. Like the French, the Belgians value their lunch hour and, most days, work paused for an hour in the middle of the day. While I didn't want to spend the whole time eating, I often took the opportunity to take a walk in the forest over the road. I came back relaxed and refreshed and I am sure that my afternoon productivity benefited as a result. Indeed, during that period, I attended a seminar where we were shown brain activity scans of a person who had been sitting down for 2 hours, and then the effect of just 20 minutes' walking. The effect was incredible. After sitting down, large parts of the brain had shut off – gone into 'sleep mode', yet after just a short walk, the brain was all lit up and firing on all cylinders.

I now make it a habit to get out into the fresh air some time every morning. I am lucky enough to live in the New Forest in southern England so I walk out with my dog and can be in open heathland with the ponies in just a few minutes. If I am at work, usually in a clinic, then I make a point of leaving the building and going out to buy a cup of coffee. Unless it is pouring with rain, I sit outside for a few minutes just enjoying being, before returning to my clinic. Just a short break outside can not only wake up the brain (thereby using up more energy so less is stored as fat), but it also helps to disrupt the constant state of stress that I would otherwise be in, helping reduce my cortisol levels – and bringing all the benefits that come with that.

A few years ago, there was some very interesting research that showed that spending two hours a week in nature is associated with better health and wellbeing. In that study, nature didn't mean being in open countryside, it also included a walk in a town park or along a riverbank.[42] The 2 hours didn't need to be taken in one go, but could be made up of several smaller periods, like my 15-minute breaks each day, perhaps with a longer walk at weekends. This effect wasn't just as a result of physical activity as it was also seen in people with disabilities. There is something calming about being surrounded by nature.

Have a think about what changes you can build into your daily routine that can reduce the risk of being constantly under stress. We cannot avoid the situations that cause us to become stressed, but we can hopefully learn to be more aware of how it makes us feel or behave. If you can recognize the symptoms, then hopefully you can take some corrective action to reduce the effect of stress on your body.

Looking after you

In a busy world, where we have to juggle work and family responsibilities, it can be easy for us to forget to look after ourselves. Yet if you have prediabetes or type 2 diabetes, it is essential that you take some time and effort to prioritize your own health. So far, we have largely focused on improving physical health. It is also important to look after our own mental wellbeing. We all need some 'me time'; a period of time on a regular basis just for you. Many of us are not very good at this. I have seen many patients over the years who prioritize the needs of their children, spouse or elderly parents over their own needs. For anyone, that can lead them to become drained and exhausted and in a constant state of stress. But if you have a health condition that requires your attention, not attending to your own needs can be positively harmful to you. Looking after you is not being selfish. After all, if we do not value ourselves enough to look after ourselves and cater for our needs, then who will? And if, as a result, something happens to us, then those dependent on us will be left to fend for themselves. So is there something that you would like to do, just for you, once or twice a week? It could be anything: an exercise class, learning a new skill, learning to play an instrument or even sitting down in front of your favourite TV programme. The only thing that matters is that it is something that gives you pleasure.

The ultimate rest is, of course, sleep and allowing ourselves to get a good night's sleep is very important. All too often, however, we squeeze sleep in only when we have finished our day's business, regardless of when that is. I mentioned that a few years ago I lived in Brussels. There I worked in an international policy role, which meant that I was in contact with people from all around the world. Consequently, emails would come in thick and fast around the clock – and right into my phone. Now you have already heard how I have mild addictive tendencies towards ice cream. My confession in this chapter is that if my phone is in my pocket, I am subconsciously always waiting for the next message to come through. Recognizing this, I have to plan specific times when I part myself from my phone, especially in the evenings, when it stays on my desk. I also have a rule to keep it out of the bedroom. However, I will often check it just before going upstairs to bed, and also first thing in the morning. Thankfully I have managed to stay away from Facebook, but a few years ago I was persuaded that I really ought to be on Twitter, and so that has now joined my phone-checking routine.

Undoubtedly, having ready access to friends and work colleagues at all times does have its benefits. But it also has its downsides. What might be the effect of receiving a work email just before going to bed? Or a non-urgent but difficult text from a family member, just as you set off for a nice evening out – or even worse, while you are out? At best, they will cause a certain amount of stress. At worst, they will make you feel you have to change your plans or stay up to deal with it, or lie awake at night worrying about it. Some companies are now realizing this, and in Germany, a number of companies have issued a ban on using work email outside of normal working hours. They recognize that employees will be far more productive during the day after a good night's sleep, than if they are up all hours responding to unnecessary emails.

Social media and other modern technology are just one cause of disturbed sleep. Some of us work in a culture where it is considered 'virtuous' to stay up until 3 am working to meet a deadline. How wrong we are. It has been shown that poor sleep has a bigger impact on driving performance than drinking alcohol. One of my trips to Bermuda coincided with a rail strike in the UK, and so I had to drive to the airport and leave my car there. This meant that I had to drive back home after the overnight return flight, in which I had had maybe, at most, two hours' sleep. The drive took about two hours but I was aware my reaction times were slowed and it was a real struggle to stay awake. Halfway home, I felt in desperate need of coffee and sugar to keep me alert. This wasn't just psychological. Poor sleep leads to increased levels of – you guessed it – cortisol, which increases appetite but decreases satiety; so you need to eat more and still feel hungry. You will not be surprised to learn that, even in people without diabetes, blood sugar levels are higher after disturbed sleep, setting off the train of insulin resistance and fat storage, weight gain and type 2 diabetes. Good sleep, on the other hand, has the opposite effect – it is incredibly beneficial.

In his book, *The 4 Pillar Plan*, Dr Rangan Chatterjee has a whole chapter on how to improve sleep, with many helpful tips. These include having screen-free time for 90 minutes before going to bed. Quite apart from the impact that stress from the emails, Twitter messages or the TV programme on the screen has in disturbing sleep, the blue light emitted from screens tricks our brains into thinking it is still daytime, disturbing the hormone changes that make us sleepy, and thus risking keeping us awake into the night. A double whammy. Instead, try purposefully relaxing and aiming (where possible) to avoid mental stress or excessive exercise in the late evening, having phone-free time and absolute darkness in the bedroom.

Diabetes distress

It has been recognized that having type 2 diabetes itself can be a cause of psychological ill health, and the term 'diabetes distress' is used to describe the emotional and psychological effects experienced by people with diabetes. Diabetes distress is associated with higher HbA1c levels, and increased risk of diabetes-related complications and so it is important that it is taken seriously.

Diabetes distress is likely to result from a number of factors that affect people with the condition. These include how individuals respond to being diagnosed with type 2 diabetes, how they adjust to the lifestyle changes required to control it, and how they cope with complications if they arise. Even in the absence of long-term complications, just having high blood glucose levels can affect mood or the ability to concentrate, as well as cause unpleasant physical symptoms, such as thirst, frequent urination and erectile dysfunction. These impacts readily explain how having diabetes can affect relationships, family life and employment. It is also easy to imagine how someone, burdened by these problems, might find it more difficult to make the necessary changes to their diet and lifestyle in order to manage their diabetes. It is not surprising, therefore, that diabetes distress is associated with being less physically active, having an unhealthy diet and being less regular in taking medications. All of which can lead to higher blood glucose levels and greater risk of the complications we discussed in Chapter 3.

A number of studies have shown that the way people are managed when they are first diagnosed with type 2 diabetes creates a significant mental impression; and it's something that stays with them for many years. Not only does it impact on a person's diabetes control and physical health, but also on their psychological health.

For many people, being diagnosed with diabetes comes as a nasty shock – and may be associated with a number of different powerful emotions. Some of these can result from the thoughts, feelings and worries that naturally emerge when you are diagnosed with a health problem. These can be compounded by the stories other people may tell you about how, for example, diabetes caused their uncle to go blind and lose both legs.

Getting the right information at the beginning can help correct any misinformation that may lead to negative emotions. Until recently, even giving accurate information may have caused negative emotions, as it was believed that type 2 diabetes was always permanent and, over time, would gradually and inevitably get worse. Put crudely, the message was, 'you will have it for life, it will get gradually worse, but you can make changes that can slow down how quickly it gets worse'. For some people, who for whatever reason may be poorly motivated or rather despondent in their outlook on life, this could lead to a feeling of, 'whatever I do won't make that much difference, so I might as well get on and enjoy myself'. We now know that type 2 diabetes can be reversed – and those who are newly diagnosed or who have prediabetes have the greatest chance of reversing the condition. To my mind, this is essential information for anyone newly diagnosed with type 2 diabetes. Knowing that diabetes can be reversed could fundamentally affect how people respond in terms of the effort they put in to making the necessary changes to their lifestyle (as described earlier in this book). It also provides a message of hope and of empowerment – that the changes you make can and will help you improve your health. If conveyed correctly, I believe that this could lead to a lot less diabetes distress arising at the time of diagnosis.

Another source of diabetes distress arises from the traditional advice about how diabetes should be managed, with its emphasis on medication rather than lifestyle, coupled with its guidance on diet that may actually make things worse. Both risk increasing feelings of helplessness. Focusing on prescribing medication can convey the message that it is the tablets that are the treatment and can reduce the potential for the person to take control of their condition, especially if that medication leads to them putting on weight. A high-carbohydrate diet risks causing high blood glucose levels, and further risks causing confusion and despondency in someone who believes they are doing 'the right thing'. I am a firm believer that a more emphatic focus on lifestyle changes as the main means of treating type 2 diabetes and prediabetes, coupled with a simple explanation about which foods will help reduce blood glucose levels, will help people feel they are in control of their condition and will reduce feelings of helplessness and of anxiety.

To summarize, having poor mental health can be part and parcel of the effect of our modern lifestyles, just as gaining excess weight or developing type 2 diabetes can be. It can also result from having diabetes. The good news is that the remedies are the same. Eating more healthily, increasing your physical activity, having rest and me time, and getting good sleep will all help improve your mental health as well as your physical health.

However, if you find that, despite making some of the changes suggested here, you still feel low in mood, then please do seek medical advice, in case you have a condition that requires specialist treatment or medication.

CHAPTER 15

Situations that require special attention: illness, stress and pregnancy

In Chapter 3, we learnt how, if you have type 2 diabetes, you are at greater risk of ill health as a result of a two-way interaction that means that diabetes affects other illnesses, and other illnesses affect diabetes. The best way to minimize this effect is to ensure your blood glucose levels are as near normal as possible, and most of this book is designed to help you achieve that, whether or not you manage to reverse your diabetes completely. However – even if you do achieve remission of your diabetes – it is important to be aware that there are some situations that might make you more insulin resistant again and cause blood glucose levels to increase. This chapter is designed to provide you with the information you need to keep yourself as well as possible, during periods of illness, stress and pregnancy.

Any situation that increases the level of glucose in the bloodstream will affect the body's functioning in two important ways: firstly, a very high glucose level can lead to dehydration and low blood pressure, which may impair kidney function; secondly, it can make you more susceptible to infection, and also for the infection then to affect you more seriously than someone who does not have diabetes. As discussed in Chapter 3, Covid-19 vividly and often tragically highlighted the increased risks associated with having diabetes. This resulted from the rather complex effects diabetes can have on the way the body fights infection, and because of the simple fact that glucose is a fuel for all living organisms.

Managing the impact of illness

As we have already discussed, keeping blood glucose levels as normal as possible will help prevent further health problems, such as eye, foot or kidney disease. It will also help ensure that, if you become ill, any effect of having diabetes will be minimized. This was again highlighted during the Covid-19 pandemic, when people with diabetes who had high glucose levels did less well than those with lower levels.

However, it is important to recognize that any illness is a stress on the body, and is associated with activation of the immune system and increased levels of stress hormones such as cortisol and adrenaline. These hormones counter the effect of insulin, causing glucose to be released from the liver into the bloodstream. Even if your diabetes is generally under very good control, any illness can cause your blood glucose levels to rise. This also applies if you have achieved remission of diabetes or prediabetes, when by definition you have achieved near-normal blood glucose levels for at least three months. The effect of stress hormones released during illness is to make you more insulin resistant. Depending on the extent to which the metabolic problems have been truly reversed, this may lead to the return of high glucose levels. While it is true that experiencing high glucose levels for a few weeks (or even months) is unlikely to lead to significant long-term damage, the high glucose levels may cause unpleasant symptoms, as well as causing the illness to take longer to resolve, especially in the case of an infection.

In a similar way, many people also experience high glucose levels after a vaccination. In a sense this is a good sign, as it indicates that the vaccine has activated the immune system, but it is understandably a cause of concern, as the effect can last for a few weeks.

As a result, it is important to recognize that your glucose levels may be higher than normal during periods of illness. Even a mild viral illness, which may cause no more than a headache and a runny nose, may have quite a profound effect on blood glucose levels. Whether you manage your diabetes with diet and lifestyle changes alone or with medication, it is especially advisable to avoid sugary or high-carbohydrate foods when you are ill. Simple fluids, ideally plain water, should be taken. Even if you do not regularly check your blood glucose, I would suggest checking it at least once a day when you're ill – for example, first thing in the morning. If the level is above 8 mmol/l (140 mg/dl), you are advised to consult your doctor in case you require medication to help control your glucose levels during the period of illness.

If you're on diabetes medication, when you're ill it may be necessary to increase it in order to control glucose levels. This could mean increasing the dose of your existing medication or starting new medication just for the period of illness. If you are admitted to hospital, your diabetes should be monitored closely and be reviewed by a member of the diabetes team, who will be able to adjust your medication in order to stabilize your diabetes control if it becomes necessary. Very often you will be able to return to your previous treatment before, or shortly after, going home again.

Illness can also cause problems with kidney function, especially in people who have a degree of diabetic kidney disease. I have already mentioned that metformin, which is one of the safest and most effective medications for type 2 diabetes, should not be used in people whose kidney function is impaired. As a rule, anyone who takes metformin or a sodium-glucose co-transporter-2 (SGLT2) inhibitor should stop taking it if they need to be admitted to hospital with an acute illness, or if they have any illness that causes dehydration, such as prolonged vomiting or diarrhoea, as these are situations that can increase the risk of affecting kidney function or causing a metabolic disturbance. If you have impaired kidney function and take medication for high blood pressure, it may be advisable to stop these during periods of illness as well. It is a good idea to discuss this with your diabetes care team in advance, so that you know what to do during periods of illness.

If you are on a sulfonylurea or insulin, the dose will need to be increased if glucose levels rise; on the other hand, if your illness means you are not eating normally, these medications could cause your blood glucose level to fall too low. In that situation, it is very important to check your glucose levels more frequently, and if levels are falling below about 5 mmol/l (90 mg/dl), the dose of sulfonylurea or insulin will need to be decreased. This is a situation where you should take medical advice on the best course of action.

In terms of other medications, as already mentioned, any blood pressure medication may need to be stopped if you are experiencing diarrhoea or vomiting that lasts more than a day, especially if your kidney function is impaired. Some medications for other conditions can also affect glucose control. The most important are steroids, usually taken as tablets such as prednisolone. This is used in high doses for people who have exacerbations of asthma and many other inflammatory conditions. If you need to take steroids, then it is possible you may also need to have insulin (or a higher dose of insulin) while you are on steroids. There are many other tablets that can potentially increase glucose levels. These include thiazide diuretics, beta blockers, antipsychotic drugs, some antibiotics and statins. Conversely, selective serotonin reuptake inhibitor (SSRI) antidepressants, such as sertraline and citalopram, can reduce glucose levels. I recommend that you read the leaflets that come with your medications to see if they could affect your glucose levels.

As a general rule, I would advise anyone with type 2 diabetes who takes medication to discuss with their doctor what they should do with each of their medications in the event of illness (both those for diabetes and those for other conditions). In this way, you can construct your own 'sick day rules' that should be kept handy, so that you can easily refer to the list if you become unwell. Table 14 provides an example.

Table 14: Sample sick day rules for someone with diabetes and taking medication

Tablet	Dose	Taken for	If I become unwell
Metformin	500 mg twice a day	Diabetes	Stop if I have diarrhoea and vomiting
Gliclazide	40 mg daily	Diabetes	Check blood sugar levels, may need to increase dose to 80 mg (check with doctor)
Ramipril	5 mg daily	High blood pressure	Stop if I have diarrhoea and vomiting
Prednisolone	30 mg for 5 days	Exacerbation of bronchitis	Increase gliclazide to 80 mg twice a day (check with doctor)

Managing the impact of stress

In Chapter 12, we discussed how life can suddenly and often without warning throw a massive spanner in the works. It could be the unexpected loss of a job, a bereavement, relationship difficulties or any other stressful life event that could lead people to deviate from their eating plan and resort to comfort foods likely to increase their blood glucose levels. It is important to be aware, however, that – even if a person does stick to their eating plan – the same factors that increase blood glucose levels during illness, such as activation of the immune system and increased levels of cortisol and adrenaline, can occur during times of stress to cause blood glucose levels to increase. Therefore, if you find that your blood glucose levels increase during a stressful period, I would recommend using some of the techniques discussed in Chapter 14 to help minimize the impact of the stressful situation on your health. Please also consult your doctor or diabetes nurse for advice as to whether you need a temporary change to your medication to help control your glucose levels, or indeed medication to help you through the stressful situation.

Pregnancy

Although pregnancy is, of course, not an illness, it has important metabolic effects that need to be taken into account. These include increasing insulin resistance in the later stages of pregnancy – which means that, if your diabetes is in remission, it may reappear at some stage during the pregnancy.

As type 2 diabetes affects increasingly younger age groups, pregnancy is now not uncommon in people with type 2 diabetes and if you are in the age group where you could become pregnant, it is important to be aware of how pregnancy might affect your diabetes and vice versa.

The key facts to be aware of are:

- It is important to achieve good and stable control of your diabetes right at the start of pregnancy, and ideally before you get pregnant. That greatly reduces the risks of any foetal abnormalities or other problems occurring during the pregnancy.

- A high dose of folic acid (5 mg daily) is recommended from the time you start to try for pregnancy.

- Certain medications should be stopped before you become pregnant, or as soon as you find out you are pregnant. These include statins, some blood pressure medications, such as ACE inhibitors, and some diabetes medications, such as glucagon-like peptide-1 (GLP1).

- It is important to check your blood glucose much more frequently, and to aim for fasting glucose levels below 5.3 mmol/l (95 mg/dl) and below 7.8 mmol/l (140 mg/dl) one hour and 6.4 mmol/l (115 mg/dl) two hours after meals.

- It is likely that you will become less insulin resistant in the first few weeks, and then more insulin resistant as your pregnancy progresses. Insulin treatment is often used in the later stages of pregnancy to achieve the required glucose levels.

- Pregnancy can affect some diabetes-related complications, such as high blood pressure, kidney disease or diabetic eye disease. It is therefore important that these are monitored during pregnancy.

It is not recommended that you make a significant change to your diet during pregnancy. If you are already on a low-carbohydrate diet when you become pregnant, then it is safe to continue during the pregnancy. As pregnancy progresses, you may experience your glucose levels increasing. A gradual reduction in your carbohydrate intake may help prevent this and reduce the need for insulin. If you are on a very low-carbohydrate, ketogenic diet, then you should advise your health carers. Some experts consider a ketogenic diet to be unsafe in pregnancy, while others consider it a safe option.[43] If nothing else, routine screening will show ketones in your urine, and this could otherwise be a cause for concern, so it is important to tell your medical team if you are on a ketogenic diet.

CHAPTER 16

The importance of regular health checks

Once you have been diagnosed with type 2 diabetes, it is important to have regular health checks performed, usually once a year, to assess whether you have any signs of impending complications that might need treatment. The aim of this chapter is to explain about each of these checks, and how you should go about getting them done.

If you have had type 2 diabetes for many years, it is likely that there will be some blood vessel disease, even if you do not have much in the way of symptoms. If you then manage to reverse your diabetes, while that will have greatly improved your overall health, and there is evidence that some of the long-term complications of diabetes can be reversed, there may still be some lasting impact from having had diabetes. While there is encouraging evidence that small vessel disease, affecting the eyes, nerves or kidneys, can improve with remission, long-term large vessel disease that has led to significant reduction in blood flow to your legs, or coronary artery disease affecting the blood supply to your heart, are unlikely to reverse. Over time, calcification can occur that essentially makes these kinds of changes permanent. It is therefore recommended that, if you do put your diabetes into remission, you continue to have these regular checks, so that any enduring impacts of the diabetes can be monitored, and treatment provided if necessary.

If you have prediabetes, eye and feet checks are not necessary but the other checks (blood pressure, cholesterol and kidney tests) are recommended.

The eyes

Eye checks are important to detect the earliest signs of diabetic eye disease. To recap, diabetic eye disease leads to abnormalities in the small blood vessels at the back of the eye. The condition can be managed, and even reversed, by good control of blood glucose and blood pressure. However, the early changes do not affect eyesight and the only way of knowing whether you have them is by having a photograph taken of your retina. In the UK, we are fortunate in having a comprehensive eye screening service, which is free of charge for people with diabetes. This is separate from the usual eye test that you might have to determine if you need glasses.

The test involves drops being put into your eyes that dilate the pupils (making them bigger) so that there is a good view of the retina behind it. You will then be asked to sit still in front of a specialized camera that takes a photograph of your retina through the pupil. The image is usually ready immediately, and in many cases the person taking it will be able to show it to you. It will then be transmitted to a grading centre, where an expert will assess it for evidence of any diabetic eye disease. In due course, you will receive a letter confirming the findings. If all is well, you will be invited back for another test after one or two years. If there is evidence of retinopathy, then a further test may be recommended in 6 or 12 months' time. In the meantime, it would be good to consider what you can do to ensure that your glucose levels and blood pressure are as near to normal as possible. If the image shows evidence of more severe retinopathy, an appointment will be made for you to see an eye specialist (ophthalmologist) who can perform a more detailed examination and discuss possible treatments with you.

Meanwhile, the most important thing you can do is just turn up for the eye test. Some people have told me how they are fearful of having the test done in case it shows some evidence of diabetic eye disease. While I can understand the quite natural fear, I would urge you not to let it stop you having the test done as – in the early stages – good control of blood glucose levels can stop retinopathy progressing, and even help reverse it. For more advanced disease, treatment is available – and this can keep it under control and protect your eyesight.

The feet

Regular foot examination is a key part of diabetes care. Feet can be affected both by diabetic nerve disease – causing numbness and loss of sensation in your feet – and by blood vessel disease that reduces blood flow. It is therefore important that your feet are examined on a regular basis (at least once a year). The examination is relatively straightforward and includes a check on the pulses in the feet (preferably using a Doppler machine that assesses the flow through the arteries) and a simple check to test sensation. A nylon fibre (called a monofilament) is used to touch the soles of the feet in specific areas to see if you can feel it. The tests may pick up problems before you are aware of them, and if they do, should prompt a review of your diabetes management to ensure that everything is being done to minimize any further damage. Usually, the team at your doctor's surgery or at your diabetes clinic carries out these tests; it does not really matter where the tests are done – the important thing is that they are done and the results acted upon.

Kidney function

Kidney function is assessed by means of blood and urine tests that should be performed once a year. The blood test measures the estimated glomerular filtration rate (or eGFR) and is a measure of kidney function. The eGFR is calculated using a formula that depends on the amount of creatinine in the blood. Creatinine is a by-product of the body's breakdown of protein and is excreted by the kidneys. If the kidneys are not working properly, creatinine is not excreted into the urine and so the amount in the blood accumulates. A normal eGFR is generally over 90, although many people may have an eGFR below this. A level below 60, however, is definitely indicative of some impairment of kidney function. The blood test should be performed at least once a year.

The other test of kidney function is a urine test to assess the amount of creatinine found in the urine, relative to a protein called albumin. While creatinine should be excreted into the urine by the kidneys, albumin is a protein found in the blood and there should only be a very small amount of it in the urine. However, in diabetic kidney disease, the blood capillaries become leaky, which means that substances such as albumin leak through into the urine. While this is not a good thing, it does provide a simple means of checking whether the kidneys are working properly. For this test, you need to provide a sample of urine that is sent to a laboratory to have the levels of albumin and creatinine measured. The result is expressed as the albumin to creatinine ratio (or ACR for short). A level of up to 3.5 is generally considered normal. If your test result is higher than this, it does not necessarily mean you have diabetic kidney disease, as there are a number of other factors that may cause a higher level (for example, a urinary infection or increased physical activity). Therefore, if the result is above 3.5, then two further urine samples should be taken first thing in the morning. Very often, these will be normal; however, if the levels are consistently raised then this suggests that the kidneys have been affected by diabetes.

A slightly raised level (e.g. up to 30) is termed microalbuminuria (literally, 'small amount of albumin in the urine'). If you are diagnosed with microalbuminuria, you will usually be prescribed medication to reduce the pressure in the kidneys. The usual treatment is an ACE inhibitor, such as ramipril, which is also used to treat high blood pressure. This, together with better control of glucose and blood pressure, can help reduce the albumin leak, sometimes to normal levels.

Higher levels of ACR are termed macroalbuminuria. This will also require treatment with an ACE inhibitor. This may not improve the albumin leak but will usually prevent further damage. Without treatment, however, diabetic kidney disease can progress to cause scarring of the kidneys, high blood pressure and eventually kidney failure. Fortunately, this is now rare in people with type 2 diabetes. However, there are no symptoms associated with albumin in the urine, and, as with the other checks mentioned in this chapter, it is vitally important to get the urine test done, so that if there is evidence of diabetes affecting your kidneys, appropriate treatment can be started in order to prevent more serious damage.

Blood pressure

Blood pressure is the level of pressure that the blood is under in the blood vessels. The cells that make up the body need glucose and oxygen (plus a variety of other substances) to function effectively. The job of the blood is to carry these necessary chemicals and nutrients to every part of the body. Blood is also the means by which hormones, produced in the pancreas and other endocrine organs, are transported to the different parts of the body, where they are needed to perform their biochemical action (in the case of insulin, enabling glucose to enter cells). So, for blood to function effectively, it needs nice clean blood vessels to flow through and it needs to be under pressure in order to flow (against the force of gravity a lot of the time). Obviously, if there were no pressure, the blood would just sit where it is, like a stagnant pool. Blood pressure comes primarily from the action of the heart – the specialized muscle that acts as a pump squeezing the blood through the arteries. The kidneys also have an important role in controlling blood pressure, by producing hormones that help control how tightly the blood vessels contract (to increase pressure) or relax (to reduce blood pressure). The kidneys also regulate blood pressure by controlling the amount of salt in the blood vessels. A higher salt content leads to more water being retained within the blood vessels, thus increasing blood pressure. Reducing the salt content lowers blood pressure. It will be obvious that diseases of either the heart or the kidneys may cause problems with blood pressure regulation – and can make an existing blood pressure problem worse.

One of the roles of insulin is to act on the kidneys to retain water and salt. Therefore, high insulin levels will keep more water and salt in the blood circulation, directly increasing blood pressure. This explains why people with type 2 diabetes and prediabetes are more likely to have high blood pressure.

A vicious circle can then develop whereby having type 2 diabetes increases the risk of high blood pressure; this combination in itself can then lead to heart and kidney problems, which can then make the blood pressure problem worse. High blood pressure increases the risk of further complications, such as a stroke or heart attack, and so it is essential that it is closely monitored in everyone with type 2 diabetes or prediabetes.

Blood pressure is measured using a machine connected to a cuff that is placed tightly around the upper arm. The machine causes the cuff to inflate until the pressure it exerts around the arm is high enough to stop the blood flowing through the main artery, called the brachial artery. The cuff pressure is then gradually decreased until the blood flow returns to normal. As it does, a sensor detects when the cuff reaches the level of the pressure in the arteries as the heart is contracting (called systolic blood pressure) and the level of the pressure as the heart is relaxing (called diastolic blood pressure). These results are then displayed on a digital display as two numbers, with the systolic pressure first – for example, 120/80. The actual numbers refer to millimetres of mercury (mm Hg), relating back to the days of manual machines that had a column of mercury in them, like a thermometer.

There are many guidelines that specify the ideal levels of blood pressure in different circumstances, but as a general rule it should be below 140/90. If you are young, or have evidence of kidney or eye disease, then a lower level may be recommended. Here, it is important to mention that, just like blood glucose, blood pressure levels vary quite considerably during the day, according to what you are doing and experiencing. Blood pressure can rise very quickly if, for example, you get a sudden shock or undertake sudden intense exercise or physical activity. Just as a single blood glucose measurement cannot give an accurate overview of your diabetes control, neither can a single blood pressure measurement be used to determine your blood pressure control.

Ideally, blood pressure should be measured in a relaxed environment after resting for at least five minutes. And yet it is very often measured in a busy clinic setting, perhaps after you have been waiting for some time, getting more and more tense. I therefore recommend that everyone with prediabetes or diabetes buys a machine for home use. These can be purchased for around £30 ($45). If your blood pressure is normal, I would suggest checking your blood pressure no more than once every two weeks – just to reassure yourself (and your doctor) that all is well. Obviously, if your blood pressure is already high, or you are on medication for blood pressure, then more frequent monitoring may be required. If your blood pressure has been found to be consistently high, then you are at increased risk of further health problems, and it is important to try to reduce it. You may need tablets to achieve this, but making lifestyle changes should also help.

First, by following the dietary changes that I recommend in this book, you will likely reduce your blood insulin levels and this should help reduce your blood pressure as well as your blood glucose levels. Stress can also increase blood pressure, and so managing stress, as discussed in Chapter 14, will also help keep blood pressure under control. Stress sometimes leads to drinking too much alcohol. While there is plenty of evidence to suggest that drinking a moderate amount of alcohol is not harmful to people's health, drinking more than the standard guidelines (14 units per week) is associated with several health problems – including a rise in blood pressure. So, if you drink more than the recommended guidelines – and beware, many of us underestimate the amount of alcohol we drink – then it is likely to be contributing to your high blood pressure, and I would recommend you consider how you might cut down. I know many people who have managed to do this quite successfully by adopting some ground rules for drinking. These might include: not drinking alcohol alone; not drinking at home; not having beer in the house; or nominating two or three days each week when you will not drink alcohol. Some people decide to stop alcohol completely for a time, while they focus on losing weight. The important thing is that whatever you decide to do is realistic and something that you can keep up.

Finally, salt increases blood pressure. This is, after all, how the body regulates blood pressure. The traditional advice has been that people with high blood pressure should reduce their salt intake. Certainly, if you have a lot of salt in your meals, then reducing it may help reduce your blood pressure. Avoiding ready meals and processed foods will automatically reduce your salt intake. However, I would place a greater emphasis initially on reducing starches and sugars to reduce your insulin level – and thereby indirectly reducing the salt in your circulation.

Cholesterol levels

In Chapter 7, I explained that I feel fat has been given a bad name. I think the same can be said for cholesterol. Just as we need fat, we also need cholesterol for many functions. Cell membranes, which control what enters into cells of the body, are largely made of cholesterol. Vitamin D, essential for healthy bones, and many hormones are also made from cholesterol. So, cholesterol is important.

However, many of us have high levels of cholesterol in our bloodstream. High levels of cholesterol have been shown to be associated with cardiovascular disease, such as heart attacks and strokes. It has also been shown that eating a diet high in saturated fat increases cholesterol levels. As we discussed in Chapter 7, this led to the belief that – as eating saturated fat increases cholesterol levels, and as cholesterol levels increase the risk of cardiovascular disease – eating saturated fat must increase the risk of heart disease. A belief that has since been challenged by many research studies.

Just as there are some types of fat that are better for us than others, there are many types of cholesterol, and they are not all bad. In fact, it is the balance of the different types of cholesterol that is important, rather than the total number. There are two main types of cholesterol, LDL (low-density lipoprotein) cholesterol (generally thought of as bad for us) and HDL (high-density lipoprotein) cholesterol, generally thought of as healthy. There is another type of fat called triglycerides, that are also generally accepted to be harmful.

As a rule, your cholesterol levels should be within the limits shown in Table 15.

Table 15: Healthy levels of cholesterol

Type of cholesterol	Healthy level
Total cholesterol	Below 5 mmol/l (190 mg/dl)
LDL cholesterol	Below 3 mmol/l (115 mg/dl)
HDL cholesterol	Above 1 mmol/l (40 mg/dl) in men Above 1.2 mmol/l (45 mg/dl) in women
Triglycerides	Below 1.7 mmol/l (150 mg/dl)
Total:HDL ratio	Below 4
Trig:HDL ratio	Below 2

The pattern most associated with heart disease is a low level of HDL cholesterol and a high level of triglycerides. Therefore, if you have high levels of HDL cholesterol and low levels of triglycerides, you are likely to have a reduced risk of heart disease, even if your total cholesterol level is high because of the high HDL level. Moreover, there is some evidence to suggest that this applies even if there is a high level of LDL cholesterol. That is why risk calculators such as QRISK3®[44], which estimate a person's risk of cardiovascular disease, use the ratio between total and HDL cholesterol rather than the absolute numbers.

Tables 16 and 17 show examples of different cholesterol patterns and illustrate that, even if the total cholesterol is high, as in examples 1 and 3, if the HDL is high and triglycerides low, this can still be a healthy pattern.

Table 16: Examples of different cholesterol patterns (mmol/l) and their risk profiles

In mmol/l	Ideal value	Example 1	Example 2	Example 3
Total cholesterol*	Below 5	6.3	4.7	9.1
LDL cholesterol	Below 3	3	3.5	4.0
HDL cholesterol	Above 1 (m) Above 1.2 (f)	1.8	0.5	3.1
Triglycerides	Below 1.7	0.7	3.2	0.5
Total:HDL ratio	Below 4	3.5	9.4	2.9
Trig:HDL ratio	Below 2	0.4	6.4	0.16
Risk		Low risk	High risk	Low risk

* There are more types of cholesterol than LDL and HDL and so the total cholesterol is more than the sum of these two.

Table 17 shows the same information for our friends in the US and other countries that use mg/dl units.

Table 17: Examples of different cholesterol patterns (mg/dl) and their risk profiles

In mg/dl	Ideal value	Example 1	Example 2	Example 3
Total cholesterol	Below 190	244	182	352
LDL cholesterol	Below 115	116	135	155
HDL cholesterol	Above 40 (m) Above 45 (f)	70	19	120
Triglycerides	Below 150	62	283	44
Total:HDL ratio	Below 4	3.5	9.4	2.9
Trig:HDL ratio	Below 2	0.4	6.4	0.16
Risk		Low risk	High risk	Low risk

When starting a low-carbohydrate diet, many people increase their intake of fats. This is especially the case for people on a very low-carbohydrate, ketogenic diet. This has led to some concern that it could result in increased cholesterol levels. Overall, this does not seem to be the case. Dr Unwin's patients (see Chapter 5) showed a reduction in their cholesterol levels on a low-carbohydrate diet. The patients in the Virta Health study showed a slight increase overall, but the main reason for this was an increase in HDL cholesterol. There was also a reduction in triglycerides, meaning that the net change was to a healthier cholesterol profile. In my patients in Bermuda, there was a slight increase in LDL cholesterol but a significant increase in HDL cholesterol, again indicating a beneficial change.

Some people experience a significant rise in their cholesterol levels when they go onto a low-carbohydrate diet. They have been termed 'hyper responders' and within the overall rise, there is generally a proportionately greater rise in HDL, and reduction in triglycerides, as in example 3 in Tables 16 and 17, indicating a healthy pattern overall.

The UK NICE guidelines suggest that people with type 2 diabetes should be offered treatment with a statin, if their QRISK3® assessment suggests they have a 10 per cent risk or greater of developing cardiovascular disease over the next ten years. This tool uses your HDL and total cholesterol levels to calculate your risk. If your HDL is too low, and consequently increases your risk, you may wish to have it repeated a few months after you have made lifestyle changes to reduce your overall risk.

The good news is that the same changes that help reduce your blood glucose and blood pressure will also help your cholesterol level. So, increasing your physical activity, eating a healthy diet and losing weight will all contribute to improving cholesterol levels. And beware of being taken in by low-fat foods, or foods that claim to reduce cholesterol levels. While there may seem to be a certain logic that says eating less fat will reduce your cholesterol level, remember that insulin is the main fat-producing hormone, and therefore reducing your carbohydrate intake will help reduce your insulin level, which will in turn enable you to lose weight – and improve your cholesterol level.

Statins are drugs that work by reducing the amount of cholesterol released from the liver into the bloodstream. They are undoubtedly effective and are generally well tolerated, and only need to be taken once a day. However, they can cause side effects, particularly when used at higher doses. The most common side effect is the reported incidences of muscle aches and pains; sometimes this can be associated with a potentially serious inflammation of the muscles known as myositis. However, as statins have become more widely used, a number of other side effects have been reported, ranging from headaches, difficulty in sleeping, joint pains and poor concentration. If you experience a new symptom since taking a statin, my advice would be to stop the statin for a few weeks. Generally, if the symptom is related to the statin, it will soon disappear after stopping the medication. It may be that you will manage better with a lower dose of the statin, or with a different statin. Occasionally, alternative types of medication may be required.

Some people feel strongly that they do not wish to take a statin. This is a personal choice, and it is of course each person's right to decide whether they wish to take a particular treatment. My approach is to assess everyone according to their situation. If you have had a heart attack, are overweight and have high blood pressure, then taking a statin is likely to protect your health in the future. If, on the other hand, you have no history of cardiovascular disease, have lost weight and your blood pressure is normal, then it is likely that a statin will at most have only a small overall benefit.

As with high blood pressure, there are no symptoms associated with having a high cholesterol level, so it is important to have a blood test done once every year to check your cholesterol levels. These can be done at the same time as the kidney blood test. Sometimes other tests will be added, such as a check on thyroid hormone levels (an underactive thyroid is a very common problem and makes it difficult to lose weight) or liver function tests. Liver tests are often abnormal as a result of fat in the liver, which we now understand is part of the problem in causing insulin resistance in type 2 diabetes. Very often, liver blood tests improve as you adopt the changes recommended in this book.

....

CHAPTER 17

Getting support

In this book, I have set out to describe how prediabetes and type 2 diabetes typically result from modern-day living that leads us to consume too much of the wrong types of food and drink and to spend too much of our time inactive. The key to reversing type 2 diabetes and prediabetes is to reverse these behaviours: specifically, to make changes to what we eat and drink, and to increase activity levels. Some people may only need to make small changes, finding they can accomplish these quite quickly and easily. For others, even making small changes may prove difficult. And for some others still, where a greater degree of change is required, they may find the task nigh on impossible. Therefore, it is so important that, as you embark on making lifestyle changes, you are supported as much as possible by the people around you, whether it is your family, your work colleagues or your diabetes team. You will also need the right information to help you plan and make the most appropriate and effective changes.

It has long been recognized that the successful management of diabetes is largely down to the individual – as pretty much everything someone does can affect their blood glucose levels. This makes it so important that anyone with diabetes receives appropriate education to teach them how best to manage their condition. Over the past 20 years, there has been a big expansion in the provision of self-management education in the UK, which is to be welcomed. Many of the education programmes were developed before the concept of reversal of diabetes was understood, and some have not adapted to this new reality. I know of one that still recommends eating starch at every meal, even though this has not been official advice for ten years now!

Most programmes provide a few sessions over a few weeks or even just on one day, which may be enough to provide information, but are unlikely to help patients with adopting the long-term behaviour changes that are needed to reverse their condition. That is why, when I designed the programme that was implemented in Bermuda, the initial six-week course was followed up with regular updates over the period of a whole year.

In the past few years, a number of online interventions have become available. One of the first was the Low Carb Program (lowcarbprogram.com), originally launched on the diabetes.co.uk website. Not to be confused with the charity Diabetes UK, diabetes.co.uk is a commercial organization that provides a platform to support people with diabetes, not just with information but also with a wide range of forums to which people can contribute. They have promoted the benefits of a low-carb approach for people with diabetes for a number of years, and in 2015 they launched the Low Carb Program, which consisted of ten videos explaining how a low-carb approach could help people manage and potentially reverse their condition. They have since published a research paper that shows how it enables people to lose weight and reverse their diabetes.[45] Over the years, it has developed into a much more sophisticated intervention with personalized health support and is available for NHS patients in certain areas.

Similar programmes designed to support people in reversing prediabetes or type 2 diabetes are provided by companies such as Changing Health, Oviva and SecondNature. In addition, many GPs have been inspired by the work of Dr David Unwin and set up programmes in their own areas to support reversal of diabetes. Some have developed comprehensive websites that provide information free of charge for anyone, not just their own patients. These include www.fatismyfriend.co.uk and www.newforestpcn. co.uk/low-carb/. A comprehensive list of useful websites can be found in Appendix A. Even if your GP's practice does not provide a specific programme, do tell your GP or practice nurse that you are making lifestyle changes with the aim of reversing your diabetes or prediabetes. They will likely be very interested to know how you get on, and to support you on your way.

Making lifestyle changes is always easier with someone else's help and support, rather than trying to do it all on your own. It can be very difficult attempting to change your diet while others in your house continue to eat the very foods you are trying to avoid. That isn't to say that everyone else should go without cakes and biscuits (although in many cases it would be good for them too!), but if they are willing to make some changes along with you it will certainly help. Or maybe you have a friend who is also keen to make changes to their lifestyle with whom you could go walking or join an exercise class or sports club, and in this way provide support for each other. Joining a slimming club or an exercise class will not only help you towards your goal, but the discipline of having to turn up every week can be a very motivating factor, especially if you will be weighed. Hopefully, you will also make new friends through such a group – another benefit from the activity.

Once you have set your goals, and decided what changes you are going to make, I recommend that you tell people around you what you have decided to do. I can understand that you might feel uncomfortable doing this, but if you have decided you will not eat cakes and biscuits, I encourage you to let your friends and family know and ask them not to offer them to you. If you do your own cooking and shopping, then you are already in control of what you eat, and you can start the process of change by buying and cooking different foods. If you rely on someone else to do this for you, it is essential that they are on board with, and fully understand, the changes you want and need to make. It is worth taking the time to explain in some detail how you plan to change your diet, so that they understand why you no longer wish to eat big portions of pasta or mashed potato, and so they don't take offence if you refuse the food offered. Just as the changes may be difficult for you, the change can be equally difficult for the person who has to start preparing different types of meals. You may like to show them the section below as a way of explaining things to them.

Information for friends or relatives

If you live with, or care for, someone with type 2 diabetes or prediabetes, then you will be aware of the many demands that the condition places on that person, and probably on you as well. The aim of this book is to help them more effectively take control of their condition in order to reverse the disease processes that cause diabetes. That statement may come as a surprise to you, because it was previously believed that, once you had type 2 diabetes, you had it for life.

This has now been shown to be untrue. Rather, we now know that diabetes results from excess fat accumulating in the liver and the pancreas, and that by making changes to a person's diet this fat can be reduced – thus reversing the progression of the disease. In many cases, this enables the person to lose weight and to reduce or stop taking diabetes medications. In some cases, the diabetes goes into complete remission.

The main problem in type 2 diabetes is that the body cannot use insulin properly. This leads to the pancreas producing extra insulin, resulting in the levels of insulin in the blood rising too high. As insulin is the main 'fat hormone', this leads to more fat being laid down in the internal organs, which makes the problem even worse.

It is known that losing weight and getting more active can help reduce insulin levels. Therefore, the key changes that need to be made are to the diet and to activity levels. Specifically, it is important to reduce the amount of carbohydrate (sugar and starch) in the diet. This is because all carbohydrates cause the level of glucose (sugar) in the blood to rise, which is what causes the release of insulin into the bloodstream. Reducing carbohydrates therefore helps directly by keeping the blood glucose level stable. Over time, insulin levels will reduce, resulting in the loss of fat from the liver. When that happens, insulin can again work more efficiently in controlling sugar levels, which in turn means the body does not release so much of it into the bloodstream, and so on, leading to a virtuous circle of positive health benefits.

So what does this mean on a day-to-day basis? Put simply, it means cutting down as much as possible on all foods and drinks that contain sugar. It also means cutting right back on bread, potatoes, rice, pasta and cereals, as these are all turned into sugar in the body.

Therefore, a person with prediabetes or type 2 diabetes is going to be helped by having only very small portions of these foods, and will benefit from having some meals with none of these foods in them at all. I realize this may be very different from what you were told in the past – that people with diabetes should eat starchy carbohydrates with every meal. Quite simply, that approach has not worked, whereas more and more people, including many who I have treated, have found that restricting carbohydrates really does help them achieve better control of their blood glucose levels.

What does that mean in practice? For a person with prediabetes or type 2 diabetes, a breakfast based on eggs or plain yoghurt is better than cereals or toast. A salad or soup with or without a small piece of bread is better than sandwiches, a baguette or a wrap for lunch. For other meals, keeping the starchy food (potato, pasta or rice) to a very small portion on the plate and eating lots of leafy green vegetables will certainly help. For snacks, a small piece of cheese, a handful of nuts or vegetable sticks are preferable to biscuits, crisps or even fruit. And for drinks, avoiding sweet drinks, including fruit juices, is essential – better to stick to diet versions, and even better still water. Unsweetened tea or coffee with a small amount of milk is also fine.

The other change that will help is increasing physical activity. This does not have to mean going to the gym but can mean using the car less, and walking or using public transport more. It can mean going for a walk every day, and, importantly, avoiding sitting down continuously for long periods of time (for example, in front of the television or at a computer). Even getting up and walking around for a few minutes every hour or so will help.

I have noticed that people tend to do very well when their partner or a close friend supports them, especially when that person joins in, making some of the same changes themselves. In many cases, their own health improves as well and that can't be a bad thing! I am sure that the person who asked you to read this will be very grateful for your help in supporting them in making these changes. Below is a summary of the recommended diet changes, and if you are interested, you will find more detailed information in Chapters 6 and 11.

Food recommendations

The focus of this advice is to reduce your intake of foods that convert to glucose in your body and to include more foods that have little impact on blood glucose levels.

- **Sugar:** All sugars (white sugar, brown sugar, honey, molasses, etc.) are directly converted to glucose in your bloodstream. They should ALL be avoided as they will all cause spikes in your blood glucose levels.
- **Starches:** White refined carbohydrates, such as bread, rolls, rice, pasta and potatoes, should be reduced or avoided where possible. Wholegrain or healthier options may be included in limited portions. Healthier options include oats, sweet potato, quinoa, brown rice and breads with wholegrains or seeds.
- **Fruits:** All fruits contain fructose, and some fruits have less of an effect on blood glucose levels than others. Best choices include small apples or pears, and all berries – blueberries, raspberries, strawberries, etc.
- **Vegetables:** The emphasis here is that MORE is better! All green leafy vegetables and salad vegetables are good choices. Include a minimum of two portions of vegetables with meals but more can be incorporated to replace starches on your plate. Try fresh cooked cauliflower, broccoli, courgette (zucchini), aubergine, cabbage and green beans in place of large portions of pasta, potato or rice. Add flavour, taste and texture to meats with tomato, mushrooms, peppers and

onions. These all have very little carbohydrate and are good sources of plant fibre.

- **Protein:** Good-quality protein sources should be included daily. All meats, chicken, fish – particularly oily fish, such as salmon, tuna and sardines – can be eaten freely. Eggs are excellent sources of high-quality protein. Highly processed meats, such as burgers, corned beef and hot dogs, should be avoided. For vegetarians, beans and lentils are a good source of protein. Some pulses, such as chickpeas, are high in carbohydrate. Better options are red beans, kidney beans and black beans.

- **Dairy:** Milk and dairy products are another good source of protein, and there is no need to switch to soy or dairy-free milks unless you are lactose intolerant. Full-fat plain Greek yoghurt makes an excellent high-protein choice for breakfast or to replace dessert. Try plain Greek yoghurt with berries and chopped walnuts or almonds for a filling breakfast or light meal. Cheese can also be eaten in moderation.

- **Fats:** Choose healthy sources of fat. Olive oil, canola oil and coconut oil can be used. You can use small amounts of butter instead of margarine. Avocados and nuts, particularly almonds and walnuts, are also good sources of healthy fats.

- **Desserts:** Desserts are usually high in sugar and can increase cravings for more sweet foods. If you have a sweet tooth, the recommended approach is to avoid having desserts, cakes and biscuits at home. Combine berries with plain Greek yoghurt or double cream or use some of the recipes in this book or in my *Low-Carb Diabetes Cookbook* for sweet treats.

- **Beverages: All sugar-sweetened beverages, including fruit juice, should be avoided completely.** Drink water, sparkling water or water infused with lemon or lime slices.
- **Alcohol:** Alcoholic beverages are full of empty calories. Beer and mixed drinks contain carbohydrate and will interfere with losing weight. Dry white wine and red wine are good options here.

Table 18 provides some examples for each meal of the day.

Table 18: Examples of healthy meals designed to help reverse your diabetes

	CHOOSE THESE...	INSTEAD OF THESE...
Breakfast	Eggs, bacon, mushrooms, tomatoes Cold meats Plain yoghurt (with berries, fruit, seeds, nuts)	Cereals Sweetened yoghurt Toast, jam
Lunch	Soup (minimize root veg) Sardines, tuna Cold meats Salad	Sandwiches Crisps
Evening meal	Meat, fish, chicken or pulses Lots of green vegetables Starch – none or small amount only	Rice, potato or pasta-based meals
Snacks	Small piece of fruit Handful of nuts or olives Hard-boiled egg Small piece of cheese Small piece of dark chocolate	Biscuits or cakes Banana Dried fruit Chocolate bars
Drinks	Tea, coffee (no sugar, black or small amount of milk only), unsweetened herbal tea Red wine or dry white wine, spirits Sugar-free mixers	Cappuccino Sugar-sweetened beverages Fruit juice and smoothies Sweet wines, beer, cider, liqueurs

CHAPTER 18

....

Be inspired

In this book, I have aimed to provide you with the tools you need to reverse your prediabetes or type 2 diabetes, primarily by making changes to what you eat and drink. To underpin some of the main messages, I have included true stories from real people who have managed to change their lifestyles and to reverse their condition. Some found it relatively easy, some had to struggle with food addictions, and some – such as Steve, who we saw in Chapter 3 and again in Chapter 12 – experienced how bereavement led to the return of some of their health problems. I hope these stories have encouraged you to believe that change is possible, and that it is feasible to achieve your goal – even if you have previously found it very difficult to stick to a new diet or to lose weight.

For each person, their journey with diabetes or prediabetes has had a profound effect on their life and their health. For some, the positive impact on their own health after adopting these lifestyle changes has motivated them to do something in turn to help others.

A few months after *Reverse Your Diabetes* was published in 2014, I received an email from a guy called Eddy, a TV director whose credits include some well-known UK programmes including, as it happens, *Casualty*. Early in 2015, he had been diagnosed with type 2 diabetes with an HbA1c of 85 mmol/mol (9.9 per cent).

Even though he had been overweight for some time, he was shocked at the diagnosis. That same day, his wife Claire found *Reverse Your Diabetes* on Amazon and ordered a copy. He put himself onto a low-carb diet and lost 23 kg (51 pounds) in weight over 16 weeks. When we met later, he said, 'Oddly, getting my type 2 diagnosis has turned out to be the best thing that's ever happened to me. I'm now healthier and fitter than any time in the last 30 years and I now take proper care of my health. A type 2 diagnosis can feel like the end of the world but if you embrace it, it could be the start of a better life.' Based on his own experiences, he felt inspired to make a documentary film about reversal of type 2 diabetes. Over a period of time, this led to him and his wife setting up group sessions in his locality in the beautiful Lake District in the north-west of England. They developed resources and information packs and planned 4 courses of 16 weeks. They placed advertisements in local newspapers and hired venues in four different locations (to include a mix of affluent and deprived areas) and waited to see who would turn up.

They did this without any direct medical input, although Eddy did enrol a couple of friendly GPs who offered advice. In total, 35 people attended the full 16 weeks and over the following 9 months, they had lost an average of 10 kg (22 pounds) in weight. All but one saw a significant improvement in their HbA1c, and a number reversed their diabetes. Others were able to reduce their medications and see improvements in other aspects of their health, such as high blood pressure, sleep apnoea or diabetic eye disease (see Steve's story in Chapter 3). Many had no idea that by making relatively simple adjustments to their diet they could reduce or reverse their diabetes. Eddy attended a meeting with local health chiefs, where some of the participants shared their stories, but, unfortunately, he could not gain their support to continue the initiative. This seems ironic, given that, despite their lack of medical training, his and his wife's efforts had had more beneficial impact on the health of their participants than anything received by them from traditional healthcare previously. Eddy has managed to keep his diabetes in remission for most of the time since. He admits that, at times, it has been a struggle and he has gone through periods of burnout. His diabetes made a temporary reappearance during the 2020 lockdown, but it has since gone back into remission.

Dan was also diagnosed with type 2 diabetes in 2015 – a diagnosis that led him not just to change his health, but also his career. I'll let him take up the story.

DAN'S STORY

I have spent my life studying and understanding why people eat what they eat and how we can use media to manipulate people to eat what we want. I ran an advertising agency that marketed junk food. That is, until I developed type 2 diabetes.

I had been having intermittent pain in my hands for two years and my GP put me through all sorts of tests but did not come up with a diagnosis. I thought it might be diabetes, so I bought myself a test kit and there was absolutely no doubt about the result. I immediately stopped consuming sugary foods and the pain in my hands went almost overnight and hasn't been back since.

My doctor confirmed that I had type 2 diabetes and said, 'We're going to give you some pills.' Pills scare me as my dad took lots of pills. He was obese and he had type 2 diabetes and gout and, after many years of pain, he died in 2005. Now here was I at 45, I was obese and I could just see myself going on the same journey as my dad: years of pain, suffering and, ultimately, an untimely death. I was very scared of those pills and said there must be another way to do this.

So, I stepped outside of my bubble in London advertising and I began to learn about the obesity crisis and the type 2 diabetes epidemic and what's causing it; I came to the realization that, in my work, I was massively part of the problem. I read about people reversing their type 2 diabetes through diet so the first thing I did was follow the recommended diet in the UK called the Eatwell Guide. I followed it but I couldn't get my blood glucose under control. I then came across the research at Newcastle University using a very low-calorie diet of 800 calories a day, essentially shakes and leaves, and I put myself on that for eight weeks. It was intense. I fainted twice and I have never fainted in my entire life. I couldn't function as a father or a boss or a husband. It was a really hard intense diet but it was effective. I lost about

15 kg (33 pounds) and my HbA1c came down from 76 (9.1 per cent) to 56 (7.3 per cent) but it was an emergency fix and not something that was teaching me to live for the long term.

Then I discovered *Reverse Your Diabetes*. It gave me incredible clarity and just all made logical sense. It provided a plan for life rather than an emergency fix. I went to my GP and said I'm going to manage this through a low-carb diet and they said, 'You can't do that. That's just a fad diet and you can't trust it.' So I put myself on a diet of 50 g of carbs a day and over a three-month period I took my type 2 diabetes into remission. My HbA1c was 37 (5.6 per cent) and I weighed 90 kg (198 pounds). When I had my blood test, the nurse phoned me up asking, 'What's happened? It's amazing!' I told them I put myself on a fad diet.

My weight has since crept up a little, but my diabetes remains in remission. My diet ranges from about 50 to 120 g of carbohydrates per day. I used blood glucose testing to see what foods I needed to cut back on and used the results to create my own list of green, amber and red foods. About twice a year, I'll do a week of intense testing and it keeps me on the straight and narrow, and stops a few bad habits that have crept in.

Some people find it very easy to change their lifestyle. Suddenly they are running Ironman marathons but for most of us it's not like that; it's a tough journey that goes on for the rest of your life and you need to invest in building the pillars of strength to keep you going. Maybe it's to see the kids grow up and have grandchildren. We need to invest in those pillars of strength that will help you when you're finding it hard. So, I try to spend five minutes each day to invest in growing those reasons to keep going. What is my pillar of strength? My dad never met my son which is a matter of great heartbreak for me, and my fondest childhood memories are when my dad would play the piano and sing funny songs and my brother and I would laugh. I visualize in my head my son sitting at the piano with my dad doing the same thing and I have spent hours thinking about it and it gives me strength.

Once I reversed my diabetes, I noticed that my back didn't hurt so much, my teeth have been so much better than for the past ten years, my skin and my guts are better. But what is really great is how much more contented I feel within and how much sharper my brain is. I became happier. I became the best version of me that I have ever been and that's because my metabolism was functioning well, for the first time in many years.

I realized that my work was part of the problem. So I closed my advertising agency and am now on a mission to share my experience with anybody who's interested in listening. I have advised the European Union, the OECD, UNICEF and the British government on the impact of advertising on people's diet. I want to use my marketing skills to benefit people's health and not harm it. I worked on Jamie Oliver's Sugar Smart project, which is a campaign to increase awareness of sugar and how little sugar healthy people should eat. I now run a project called Veg Power to encourage children to eat more vegetables because getting kids to eat healthier foods is key to improving the nation's health.

Liz was diagnosed with type 2 diabetes in 2017 when she was 65 years old. Prior to that, her health was generally good, although she had been on treatment for high blood pressure and high triglyceride levels. She had been overweight since she was a child, and whenever she lost weight previously, it always crept back on again. Despite this, she remained active and ran her own business.

LIZ'S STORY

When I was diagnosed with type 2 diabetes, I weighed 90 kg (198 pounds) and my HbA1c was 68 (8.4 per cent). I was advised to follow a low-fat high-carb diet and prescribed metformin, although I never took it. I had heard that diabetes could be put into remission and read Michael Mosley's book, *The 8-Week Blood Sugar Diet*. I followed this low-calorie approach for three months and lost 19 kg (42 pounds) in weight to achieve remission with an HbA1c of 35 (5.4 per cent). I increased my calorie intake but stayed on a low-carb diet of around 50 g per day. I stopped having breakfast and aimed to eat within an eight-hour window each day. I continued to lose weight and now weigh 65 kg (143 pounds) – a total weight loss of 25 kg (55 pounds). My diabetes is still in remission with an HbA1c of 33 (5.2 per cent). My lipid levels have also improved and I have been able to stop my fenofibrate and statin. I have also reduced my blood pressure medication significantly.

I did not find it difficult to follow the diet. I adapted my meals and enjoyed what I was able to eat. I did miss good bread and pasta (having lived in Italy for 11 years), but considered my health was more important so have managed to stay off them. I do have a very occasional dessert as a treat and find that my blood glucose stays stable, which really does suggest my diabetes has reversed.

However, the diabetes nurse was furious! She said I should follow her advice, but once I was in remission, she was begrudgingly congratulatory. I feel that my mental and physical health has improved greatly. I have more energy and am pleased to be on much less medication. I feel so much better and have a much healthier outlook. Having been a fat child, I never imagined I could not be overweight.

———————————————————

Liz joined several online forums and met others who have been on a similar journey. Through online contacts, she joined the Public Health Collaboration (PHC), which is dedicated to informing and implementing healthy decisions for better public health (see www.phcuk.org for further information). She became a local PHC ambassador to help inform people at a local level about healthier lifestyles. This led her to set up low-carb groups for people with type 2 diabetes, referred from a local GP practice. She does this as a volunteer. She has a one-to-one chat with every person and they are then invited to join eight sessions to support them in changing their diet. Out of the 16 people in the first group, 12 achieved remission of their diabetes. There are now over 200 people on her local low-carb Facebook group, who support each other.

MARK'S STORY

In 2005, Mark left his job at a bank to become a self-employed financial adviser. He feels that the stress of the job, combined with his already unhealthy lifestyle, contributed to the diagnosis of type 2 diabetes in 2010 when he was just 39. At that time, he weighed 102 kg (225 pounds). He says, 'I felt sluggish, overweight, tired and just felt run down. I had symptoms of diabetes such as repeated thrush and a tingly foot. I didn't realize how bad I felt though until I got better.'

When he was diagnosed, he was advised to follow the Eatwell Guide and lost weight, probably because he cut out all the unhealthy takeaways. He also threw himself into long-distance running, joining the local Parkrun and doing the Great South Run, a 10-mile (16-km) road race in Portsmouth, every year. The running, together with medication, appeared to keep his weight and blood sugar under control until 2016, when they both started to increase again. He was told that his condition was progressing, and he would need to increase his medication.

All changed, however, when he happened to hear Dr Michael Mosley being interviewed on the radio. Dr Mosley explained that people with diabetes have been advised to eat the wrong foods, and that it was these foods that were leading to the condition being chronic and progressive. 'As I'd been threatened with more drugs, I felt I had nothing to lose. I bought *The 8-Week Blood Sugar Diet* and gave it a go. I cut out all bread, pasta, rice and sugar. No more breakfast cereals and no potatoes with my dinner. I started cooking too which was a first for me. I realized that preparing meals isn't as difficult as I thought, and I enjoyed the reward of eating what I'd cooked rather than putting a ready meal in the oven for 20 minutes. The changes in my weight and blood sugar levels were very quick. I didn't find it too hard. I can be tempted to eat the wrong things and if out with friends I wouldn't get too anxious over what I ate, but I wouldn't let that allow me to "fall off the wagon" for days on end. I'm lucky like that but I think you need to know yourself and whether you can have the odd thing without undoing all your good work.'

He lost nearly 20 kg (44 pounds) in weight and his diabetes is now in remission. He feels much better, both mentally as well as physically. 'In 2018, I was invited by Dr David Unwin to speak in the UK Parliament alongside medical experts to discuss reversing diabetes. If you had asked me previously to stand up in front of audiences or push myself forward like that, I would have avoided it and thought of any reason to get out of it. My confidence just wasn't there. I feel like a fog lifted from my head in 2016 and I now find myself doing all manner of things and I absolutely love it. I put this down to how I now feed not only my body but my brain too.'

Mark also became an ambassador for the PHC and this has opened many doors to help others put their type 2 diabetes into remission. For the past year, he has been working with his local Primary Care Network to put on a low-carb programme for patients which, combined with movement, combating stress and prioritizing a good night's sleep, has led to some wonderful outcomes. 'So far 77 people have gone through the programme and the first 20 patients lost an average of 9 kg (20 pounds) in weight and reduced their HbA1c by 19 (1.8 per cent). It is truly heart-warming to see how happy people are, now they have a plan that works. I have just been appointed as a Health and Wellbeing Coach and I'm now an employee of the NHS. I never would have believed it!'

Whereas Liz and Mark are helping people with type 2 diabetes change their lifestyle, Josephine's journey has led her to improve the training of health professionals about the benefits of a very low-carbohydrate, ketogenic diet.

JOSEPHINE'S STORY

I live in Germany, close to the Austrian border. I am an architect and was diagnosed with type 2 diabetes in 2014 at the age of 61. In the years before I was diagnosed, I gained weight despite trying many different diets. I also had fatty liver, acid reflux, gout, high blood pressure and a high cholesterol level. I experienced fatigue and muscle pain and had difficulty sleeping. I became depressed because of constant exhaustion and pain. At one point I was diagnosed as having a psychosomatic stress disorder and offered psychotherapy. I needed a small suitcase to carry all my medications.

When I was diagnosed with type 2 diabetes, my endocrinologist told me that I was at the point of no return, and as I was unable to lose weight, I would need to start insulin injections. He said that diet was not a problem for type 2 diabetes and that I can eat whatever I like, as long as I inject the correct amount of insulin. I was advised to eat a balanced diet with lots of wholegrains, fruits and vegetables and to reduce meat, fat and salt. Not one word about reducing carbs or sugar.

I was in shock. I panicked because I watched my grandfather and my father-in-law die from diabetes and I knew about its horrifying consequences. I searched the internet for a solution. I came across a lecture by Dr Andreas Eenfeldt, the founder of dietdoctor.com. I also found Dr Eric Westman in the US and followed his advice to reduce carbohydrates to 20 g per day and to eat lots of eggs, meat and natural fats.

When I told my endocrinologist, he admitted that he had never heard of a diet that could put type 2 diabetes into remission. When I described the details, he just said, 'Well, considering your cholesterol level, if you follow this diet you will drop dead within a very short time!' But I was desperate and said, 'This is exactly why I need your help: please monitor me very closely while I am trying this diet and give me a warning shortly before I drop dead! If there is no success after six months, I will follow your advice and start insulin.' However, within three months, my diabetes was in remission and after six months I was off all my medications, apart from thyroid hormone. There was no longer any sign of chronic kidney disease, fatty liver or gout!

My family and friends didn't understand what I was doing. Some were curious and early on I tried to convince them of the benefits of a ketogenic diet. Then my son said, 'You have to stop. No one likes to listen to your keto stuff anymore. Let them get sick and eat whatever they want! We will show you how to use Twitter – so you can save the world and leave us in peace!' So, I turned to Twitter and met exceptional scientists, experts and doctors from all over the world and made many new friends – all interested in the low-carb approach.

We love to cook with real food and lots of good-quality butter, olive oil and cream that simply makes every dish delicious. Even our friends like my husband's keto bread and everybody loves my low-carb version of my Grandma's Potato Salad, using cauliflower instead of potatoes. There are only three items that I miss, because I haven't discovered any real substitute for Bavarian pretzels, pizza and pasta! We therefore decide to cheat on our diet and enjoy each of these once a year. Each time, I very quickly go back to my diet plan, which is not hard at all because I simply feel so much better.

Apart from reversing my diabetes, changing my diet has freed me from constantly craving or thinking about food. It has enabled me to regain my health. I have discovered that I am responsible for my wellbeing and health and that my body is not my enemy but a forgiving and helpful friend. I have also learnt that – even against all odds – change is possible.

Josephine found her journey difficult, not because of the diet itself, which she found easy to follow and delicious, but because of the misinformation that is still out there, especially in the German-speaking parts of Europe. She was shocked to discover that most doctors learn very little about nutrition and its impact on human metabolism, and that nutritionists and dietitians are still taught that people with diabetes should follow a low-fat diet. To help change this, she founded the Keto Live Project in 2016. Her mission is to improve knowledge about ketogenic diets to prevent and treat type 2 diabetes and other conditions. In 2019, she developed training for doctors, dietitians and other healthcare professionals, and held an international conference, bringing together experts from Europe and across the world (see www.keto-live.com). She has even persuaded me to brush up on my German and explore providing training to German-speaking health professionals on low-carb management of diabetes!

David works as a design engineer in the motorsports industry, where he is a well-known figure and regularly appears in online videos that are seen by hundreds of thousands of people worldwide. He lives in the UK and travels widely.

DAVID'S STORY

I was diagnosed with type 2 diabetes in 2011 when I was 37. Leading up to then, I had become very overweight. I had back problems, skin problems, sex problems and generally hated my life. When I was diagnosed, I weighed 150 kg (331 pounds) and my HbA1c was 97 (11 per cent). My doctor gave me a warning that he wasn't going to be able to help me if my life continued along the path it was heading. He gave me a very stern talk, but in regard to nutrition, I was told nothing. Just told to change my path. I left feeling insulted.

I went onto metformin tablets and treatment for erectile dysfunction but otherwise not much changed. However, I thought I should go to the gym to lose some weight and after several failed attempts, eventually plucked up the courage to go through the door. I started doing spinning sessions and during one session I collapsed and was unconscious. When I came round, I had pains in my chest. I drove myself to hospital, where I was diagnosed as having had a heart attack. That was in 2018.

While in hospital, I read Dr Aseem Malhotra's book, *The Pioppi Diet*, and thank God I did. Straight away I cut my carbs to 50 g per day and increased my intake of fat. I also watched YouTube videos of Dr Paul

Mason and Ivor Cummins, who provided additional inspiration for regaining my health.

I didn't find it difficult as the food was amazing and I no longer felt so hungry. I simply ate when I was hungry and stopped having snacks. I do miss the odd pizza and ice cream, but I make my own low-carb items these days. I was eating a lot of salads but began to experience excruciating abdominal pains. I gradually excluded most vegetables from my diet and the pains went. Within 14 months I had lost 55 kg (121 pounds) and my HbA1c was 30 (4.9 per cent). I now follow mostly a carnivore diet and, on most days, I eat within an eight-hour window. About once a week, I fast for 24 hours. After a few years, I weighed 83 kg (183 pounds) and had an 81-cm (32-inch) waist. Down from 150 kg (331 pounds) and a 122-cm (48-inch) waist. I no longer take any medication. My doctor was stunned. He could not believe it.

My wife also followed a low-carb diet and has also lost a lot of weight and is very happy. Friends and family now reach out and ask for help. My work involves appearing in a lot of trade videos that are seen by people all over the world. They can see that I have lost a lot of weight and very often they contact me for advice. I recommend that they get a continuous glucose monitor and look at the effect of their meals on their glucose levels. Then I suggest they change what they eat until the monitor shows their glucose is stable, or 'Eat to the flat line' as I put it. It's been a game changer for over 100 people now. Many have lost a lot of weight, and some have reversed their diabetes too. I feel great and am really pleased that I have also helped other people in trouble with their life.

For each of these people, changing their own health has led them to do something concrete that has helped many others improve their health too, or in Josephine's case, the health of their patients. It is a case of 'changed lives change lives'. Yet none of them had any form of medical or healthcare training. In the UK, there are many other examples, where non-medical people are filling the gap to provide effective lifestyle advice that people are not getting through traditional health services. I hope that their stories will not only inspire you to continue with your own journey to better health, but maybe will inspire you to help others too.

CHAPTER 19

Achieving your goals and celebrating your successes

Throughout this book, we have used real stories from real people to show how they have reversed their prediabetes or type 2 diabetes. From these stories, you will see that some people made a lot of changes all in one go, while others made more gradual changes. Some included intermittent fasting, others did not. Some adopted a very low-carbohydrate diet, others used more moderate carbohydrate restriction. At the end of the day, what matters is that they found a way to achieve their goals and now you too can find an eating pattern that helps you achieve your personal goals. As many people have mentioned, blood glucose testing is extremely helpful, and many people find success by 'eating to the meter', or as David, who we met in the last chapter, put it, when using a continuous monitor, 'eating to the flat line'. The aim is that your meals enable you to maintain stable and normal glucose levels; any that do not, need to be changed. Unless, like Josephine, who also shared her story in the last chapter, you enjoy a special occasion with one of your favourite high-carb meals (as long as it is only a very few times each year!).

How much carbohydrate you can tolerate is very individual. In my experience, some people find they can eat a moderate amount of one type of carbohydrate – for example, a type of bread – and their body copes with it quite well, whereas if they eat a different form, such as rice, their glucose level shoots up. Only by testing can you identify what types of foods your body can manage, and therefore the type of eating pattern that will be most effective for you.

The aim of this book has been to give you the information, the guidance, the support and the motivation you need to reverse your prediabetes or type 2 diabetes. Other people, books and websites can give you more information and support but actually making the changes is up to you. If you have gained a lot of weight over recent years, losing it may seem daunting, but remember, you do not have to lose a lot of weight in a short time. Your weight gain, and your diabetes or prediabetes, has likely developed over many years – like Rome, it wasn't built in a day! Remember the advice about goal-setting, to help you really identify what it is you want to achieve. Once you have that overall goal, try to split the process of achieving it into more manageable, bite-size goals.

Achieving your goals

If your overall goal is to lose weight, how much weight do you need to lose? Again, this is up to you. But if your goal is to reverse type 2 diabetes, then the research suggests that you are likely to need to lose around 15 kg (33 pounds) in weight.[46] However, if you weigh around 75 kg (165 pounds) or less, you may only need to lose around 5–10 kg (11–22 pounds) in weight. A good guide is to aim for your weight when you were in your mid-twenties (unless, of course, you were already overweight by then).

I won't deny that, if your overall goal is to lose 15 kg (33 pounds), that can seem a very huge ask. But if you break it down into smaller goals of 5-kg (or 11-pound) chunks, it becomes more manageable. Your focus is then on achieving your first goal of losing 5 kg (11 pounds). With a little willpower and determination, that could be achieved in just a few weeks. And that's a goal met!

It is important that you have some way to monitor your progress towards your goals. For monitoring weight loss, I strongly recommend that you invest in a good set of weighing scales. Digital scales are often easier to read. It also makes sense to weigh yourself at the same time of day. I generally suggest weighing yourself first thing in the morning, naked, before you have eaten anything and after you have been to the toilet. Remember that a full stomach or bladder or clothes will all increase your weight. It is generally advised to weigh yourself once a week. It's not really important how often you weigh yourself – some people like to weigh themselves every day as part of their routine – but the main thing is that weighing yourself periodically helps you identify whether you are still on track and will encourage you to achieve your goal.

Another very useful way of monitoring your progress is to measure your waist. Your lifestyle changes are designed to help you lose excess fat in your abdomen, and so as that fat reduces, your waist will shrink. Indeed, one of the most common complaints I hear is people saying they have to buy new trousers! To measure your waist, you cannot rely on your trousers' waist measurement. You need to use a tape measure and measure across the widest part, usually at the level of your tummy button. When measuring, ensure the tape measure is not too tight, and take the measurement when you have gently breathed out. Many people find that their waist is shrinking, even if they have not lost much weight.

If you have chosen to set yourself an overall goal of reducing your blood glucose levels from a high level to a much lower one, consider setting an interim goal. If your fasting glucose is generally between 15 and 20 mmol/l (270–360 mg/dl), perhaps set a goal to achieve a level of 10 mmol/l (180 mg/dl) in the first instance and measure your fasting glucose at least once a week so you can track your progress towards this mini goal.

You may well find that you achieve your first goal relatively quickly and easily, but that progress thereafter starts to slow. It can be quite disconcerting to stall after such a promising beginning, but it is an entirely normal part of the process, and there are a number of reasons for this. In respect of weight, it is quite common to lose a few kilos or pounds very quickly, because when you use up your glycogen stores, you also lose water. Weight loss then slows down, when you then start to burn fat. Similarly, if you cut out sugary foods and drinks, you will likely see a rapid drop in your blood glucose levels, but the drop might then slow down as you make further, less drastic changes. If you experience a stall in either weight loss or reduction in glucose levels, then above all, do not lose heart. It is, as I have said, entirely normal and to be expected. At this stage, it is time to have a think about whether any of the following apply in your situation:

1. Are you measuring your waist? Quite often waist circumference continues to fall, even if weight loss slows down.

2. Have you allowed any foods or drinks to slip back into your routine? Perhaps because you thought you were doing so well and could allow yourself to return to them – if so, cut them out again.

3. Are you sure there are not any 'hidden carbs' in some of the foods you are eating? Check things like sauces, salad dressings, and tinned or ready meals.

4. Are you still checking your blood glucose level before and two hours after one meal each day? If you often find the level increases after eating, do you need to reduce your carb intake further for some of your meals?

5. Are you using cheese or nuts as snacks? Remember that, while these will have very little effect in raising your blood glucose levels, their high fat and calorie content could be slowing down weight loss. Therefore, consider doing without them for a while, or at least being stricter about the amount you actually eat.

6. Are you eating too much fruit? Again, consider limiting fruit to a small portion of berries, or stopping altogether for a while, to see if this helps.

7. How much alcohol are you drinking? Remember that alcohol in any form contains 'empty calories' and has a similar effect as sugar in leading to fatty liver. That is before considering the impact of any carbohydrate in some drinks – such as beers and ciders. Can you cut out alcohol for a while?

8. Are you limiting sedentary time and building more walking into your daily routine? If not, now might be a good time to do so.

9. Are you on insulin or a sulfonylurea? If so, discuss with your doctor whether you would benefit from reducing the dose further.

Going through this list might highlight one or two changes you can make that will get you back on track. If, despite making these changes, you still feel that you are stalling, then it may be worth seeing a dietitian who can review what you are eating and provide some specific advice, personalized to you. Alternatively, or in addition, you may wish to consider introducing intermittent fasting into your routine, such as missing breakfast on a regular basis so that you have a 16-hour fast a few times a week. If you are already doing this, would you consider a 24-hour fast by having just one meal on one or two days each week? Have another look at Chapter 10.

Maybe you feel you have done all the right things but have struggled to keep the changes going. Might it be that you are addicted in some way to certain foods? If so, do you need to plan to avoid certain trigger foods completely? Have another look at Chapter 12. Or maybe you have been in a routine for so long, it just seems too difficult to change. When I was a student, I was told that once you reach the age of 30 (which at the time seemed a long way off!), our routines are so ingrained in us that it is very difficult to change them. My own experience in the many years since then leads me to believe that, while there may be a kernel of truth in the idea, we are not pre-programmed and destined never to change. After all, the way in which so many people worldwide have changed their eating behaviours – for all the wrong reasons having been encouraged to do so by highly sophisticated advertising and other marketing influences – to cause such ill health, proves that we can and do change, given the right (or wrong) stimulus.

As I have repeatedly said, reversing your prediabetes or type 2 diabetes will require you to make significant changes to your lifestyle – for the benefit of your health. Since March 2020, people all around the world changed habits of a lifetime – for the benefit of their health. I am writing this nearly 18 months later and, for much of that time, I have had to keep physically distanced from almost everyone else in the world; literally overnight, changing lifelong habits. No shaking hands, hugging, kissing or other forms of physical contact. Suddenly, what were generational societal norms became abnormal. So much so that when a friend put his hand out to shake my hand a few weeks ago (once it was permitted once more), I felt as though my personal space had been violated. In a similar way, we need to change long-held habits and attitudes about foods and drinks that are harmful to us. The changes we were obliged to incorporate into our daily lives to help combat Covid-19 compelled the whole machinery of government and the media to change, and together they mobilized to enforce our adoption of those changes, which were backed up by new liberty-curtailing legislation. The health of the nation was threatened. In contrast, it is such an irony that governments do not consider it similarly necessary to mobilize their huge powers to limit the harm done by so many of the foods and drinks that are marketed to us so relentlessly. This means that, unlike Covid changes, the changes you need to make to improve your health really are down to you. And, as you make them, you will need to contend with the full force of the food and marketing industries that will at every turn try to get you to eat and drink their harmful products.

Now adapting to a global pandemic and changing your diet are, of course, very different things, but I mention it because everyone, even those who would have said 'I can never change', had to make some changes during the pandemic. Can you learn from how you adapted to Covid in order to help you adapt to a healthier way of eating? I recall that when mask-wearing became mandatory in shops, I found myself about to go into a shop without one on several occasions, so I had to make it a habit; to make sure that whenever I left the house, I had a mask with me. There followed a few more maskless outings, making me realize I needed prompts to help me change my behaviour. We put some masks on the table near the front door and also in the glove compartment of my car. Looking back now I can see how, within a relatively short time, wearing a mask became normal behaviour. And like me, you too will have changed your behaviour. Maybe, like me, you also needed prompts to get you there. So, whether it's putting a note on your fridge, or by the biscuit tin, or avoiding going into certain shops, have a think about what you can do to help you make the lifestyle changes you need to make to improve your health and how to make them stick.

Celebrating your successes

The second part of this chapter is about 'celebrating your successes'. I have chosen the word 'successes' – in the plural – deliberately. I encourage you to celebrate every success, however small. It could be your first fasting glucose below 10, or your first day without a sweet treat. Of course, you need to be careful how you celebrate so that, in celebrating, you do not undo the progress you have made towards your goal. And don't be shy about each success. Tell a close friend, or if there's no one to hand, tell your dog. Better still, give your dog a special long walk so you can celebrate together. Try to make your celebrations unrelated to food and, above all, make the celebration something that will give you pleasure.

You may want to save an extra special treat for when you have accomplished your main goal, such as achieving remission of your condition.

So, let's recap how you can know if you have achieved remission, which is based on your HbA1c level (see Chapter 2):

- Remission of prediabetes occurs when you have achieved an HbA1c level of less than 42 mmol/mol or 6.0 per cent and kept it below that level for at least three months, without any diabetes medication.
- Remission of type 2 diabetes occurs when you have achieved an HbA1c level of less than 48 mmol/mol or 6.5 per cent and kept it below that level for at least three months, without any diabetes medication.

You will see that if you have type 2 diabetes, are able to come off all your diabetes medications and bring your HbA1c down to, say, 44 mmol/mol (6.2 per cent) and keep it at that level for at least three months, then you have achieved remission from diabetes but you still have prediabetes. That in itself is an awesome achievement and will protect you from much ill health. However, some people believe that they have only truly reversed their diabetes when they have achieved a 'normal' HbA1c level (i.e. less than 42 mmol/mol or 6.0 per cent (less than 39 mmol/mol or 5.7 per cent in the US)). Others will make significant progress with losing weight and improving their blood glucose levels, but still have diabetes. Remission is harder to achieve if you have had type 2 diabetes for many years, as some of the changes in your pancreas become permanent over time and cannot be reversed. However, in such cases, where you're losing weight while still having type 2 diabetes, your lower glucose levels and possibly decreasing need for medication still represent a huge achievement in improving your health, especially if you can keep those changes up into the longer term. Every kilogram or pound of weight lost and every reduction in HbA1c is an achievement worthy of celebration.

This chapter is designed to send you off with excitement about what you can achieve. However, I do feel it is important to emphasize a crucial fact: just as prediabetes and type 2 diabetes are reversible, remission is also reversible. That means that – if you let up on your new way of eating, and especially if you regain weight – then there is a real chance you will push your HbA1c back up and into the range for prediabetes or type 2 diabetes. The most dramatic example I have seen of this was with a gentleman who had had type 2 diabetes for over 20 years and had been on insulin for many years. His goal was to come off insulin. Within two months of starting a low-carbohydrate diet, he had not only come off insulin, he had also reduced his HbA1c into the prediabetes range. He kept it there for over six months and so, by definition, he had put his diabetes into remission. The next time I saw him was a couple of weeks before Christmas. His HbA1c had gone up to 65 mmol/mol or 8.1 per cent, meaning that his diabetes had come back. What had happened? No major life event or crisis, no bereavement. What had happened was Christmas – or rather the run-up to Christmas. He came from the US and so his celebrations had started with Thanksgiving in late November, and then as Christmas was approaching, he allowed himself to attend a few functions, and enjoy some of his favourite Christmas sweet treats. His remission had reversed – after just a few weeks of relaxing his diet.

This emphasizes the importance of sticking to your new way of eating for the long term, and continually monitoring your blood glucose levels, especially if you enjoy the occasional treat of a food you have otherwise given up. The story also highlights the importance of continued follow-up with your GP, including blood tests, at least once a year, so that you can confirm that you remain in remission. There is now a specific code used by the NHS to document 'diabetes in remission' in a patient's record to enable such checks to continue.

Earlier I said that reversing prediabetes or type 2 diabetes requires you to make significant changes to your lifestyle. We have discussed how that means you will need to make changes to routines or behaviours in relation to food that may have been with you for many years. It will also require you to 'unlearn' the myths that I outlined earlier in the book. In finishing, let us remind ourselves of the seven diabetes myths and why I believe them to be just that, myths to be discarded.

Myth 1: You have diabetes because you are lazy and eat too much.
Fact: Type 2 diabetes is rising across the world as lifestyles adapt to changing environments.

The most dramatic change has been to our food environments, where junk food has supplanted real, fresh produce, where the sustained activities of international food companies have shifted global populations towards eating a highly processed, high-calorie, carb-rich diet, leading to an epidemic of prediabetes and type 2 diabetes. You, individually, will have to learn how to recalibrate your eating habits. But be warned, the might of industrial-level marketing of the food industry will be pitched against you.

Myth 2: Prediabetes leads on to type 2 diabetes, which is an inexorably progressive condition that requires progressively more medication and eventually insulin to control it.
Fact: Both prediabetes and type 2 diabetes can be reversed through lifestyle change.

It means stopping medications, not increasing them. That might be bad news for the pharmaceutical industry, but great news for everyone who has managed to stop their medication.

Myth 3: There is no such thing as a diabetic diet – just eat healthily.
Fact: Making dietary changes is the natural way to reverse prediabetes and type 2 diabetes.

Prediabetes and type 2 diabetes are conditions in which the body cannot tolerate carbohydrates. Key to all the successful and evidence-based approaches to reverse them is a focus on reducing

313

the intake of sugars and starchy foods. That means ignoring some of the official dietary guidance that is still out there.

Myth 4: Cheese is full of saturated fat and you shouldn't eat it.
Fact: Saturated fat isn't all bad. Better to eat cheese than a biscuit.

There is plenty of evidence that saturated fat is not the enemy we were told it was, and that dairy products, especially fermented ones such as cheese and yoghurt, are positively good for us. They are minimally processed foods that are naturally low in carbohydrate, and high in protein and healthy fats. That's why it's better to eat cheese than a biscuit.

Myth 5: People with type 2 diabetes do not need to check their blood glucose levels.
Fact: Checking your blood glucose levels is invaluable for everyone with type 2 diabetes.

It is the only way that you can track your progress towards reversing your type 2 diabetes, and the only way you can check that the foods you are eating are keeping your blood glucose levels stable.

Myth 6: You need to exercise to lose weight.
Fact: Exercise is not the answer. Just walk more and sit less.

Exercise is good for your heart, your muscles and your mind. But it is no good for losing weight and will not reverse prediabetes or type 2 diabetes. Some types of exercise increase blood glucose levels and intensive exercise can be dangerous if you are unfit. However, walking more and sitting less can really help reverse the diabetes disease process.

Myth 7: You must eat three meals a day.

Fact: You don't need to eat if you are not hungry – missing meals can be good for you.

Far from being the most important meal of the day, breakfast breaks our overnight fast. Missing breakfast is a simple form of intermittent fasting which has many health benefits, including reducing insulin levels and thereby helping to reverse the diabetes disease process.

Finally, I would like to thank you for reading this book. It is my hope that it will help you take yourself to a healthier future, whether or not you manage to reverse your diabetes or prediabetes. The next section of the book contains a selection of recipes for delicious low-carb meals to help get you started on your journey.

If you do find this book helps you achieve your goals, please do write and let me know. You can contact me via my website at www.drdavidcavan.com. Maybe your story will one day inspire someone else.

PART FOUR

Recipes

About the Recipes

I said at the outset of this book that for the first 20 years or so of my career I focused on advising medication first and foremost to help people achieve good control of their diabetes. But not always with the success they and I hoped for. Then, a little over ten years ago, I started to recognise that what people eat, day-to-day, had a far greater bearing on blood glucose levels than many medications. I realised that the officially recommended low-fat, high-carbohydrate diet was a big part of the problem and it was contributing to excess weight gain and high blood glucose levels. So, I started to advise that people adopted a low-carbohydrate, healthy-fat diet – as I have explored at length in this book.

Following the publication of my first book, *Reverse Your Diabetes: The Step-By-Step Plan to Take Control of Type 2 Diabetes* (Vermilion 2014), I soon started receiving reports from people who had cut the carbohydrates in their diet and seen great improvement in their overall health and wellbeing as a result. You will have read some of their stories in this book. The benefits of such a nutritional regimen, which shares some similarities to the Mediterranean diet, are not merely confined to those with type 2 diabetes. In fact, a low-carb, healthy-fat approach to eating can result in noticeable improvements in blood pressure, weight loss (particularly reduction in belly fat), liver function and cholesterol and triglyceride levels. According to Dr David Unwin, the evidence is that these improvements can occur at any age; those over 60 years old will see as much improvement in their metabolic health as younger people.

Highly refined carbohydrates contribute to the development of type 2 diabetes, so removing them from anyone's diet is extremely effective at preventing prediabetes progressing to 'full-blown' type 2 diabetes. If you're gaining weight and at risk of developing prediabetes later on, then adopting a low-carb, healthy-fat approach to food will help. It has also been shown to help enable people with type 1 diabetes achieve stable glucose control on less insulin, which means a decreased risk of hypos and, again, a lower risk of unwanted weight gain. In fact, my co-author of *The Low-Carb Diabetes Cookbook* (Vermilion 2018), Emma Porter, has type 1 diabetes and has significantly improved her wellbeing through following a low-carb, healthy-fat approach to her diet. I recommend you have a look at her website, thelowcarbkitchen. co.uk, where you will find plenty of her fabulous recipes. Emma has kindly supplied a low-carb trifle recipe for this book (page 361). There follow approximately 30 low-carb, healthy-fat recipes that should appeal to most tastes.

What is at the heart of a low-carb, healthy-fat diet? Well, as just a small bowl of rice can raise your blood sugar by the same extent as ten teaspoons of sugar, it makes sense to avoid not only sugar but also starchy carbs, replacing them with green vegetables and more protein in the form of meat, fish, dairy products and nuts. This approach to food intake forms the heart of the low-carb diet.

Right at the start of the book in my first aid guide to taking control of type 2 diabetes, I advised you to avoid sweet foods such as cakes, biscuits, jam, sweets or chocolate; eat less potato, rice, pasta and bread; and eat more fresh green and salad vegetables. So, these recipes are designed to avoid such refined carbohydrate-loaded foodstuffs, but not at the expense of ease of preparation or tastiness. One good example is to compare Katie Caldesi's Pizza al Taglio (page 331) with a shop-bought dinner-plate-sized variety that contains 26 ingredients, many of which have ghastly sounding scientific names, and which weighs in at 75 g of carbohydrate, whereas Katie's has fewer than a dozen ingredients and results in only 3–4 g of carbohydrate per serving – and tastes all the better for it.

Speaking of Katie, I urge you to have a look at her and her husband Giancarlo's low-carb cookbooks, which I've listed in the Appendix in Further Reading (page 366). Katie has generously supplied seven new recipes for this book, plus her publisher, Kyle Books, has kindly allowed us to reproduce her pizza recipe along with four other family meals that have won considerable acclaim. Giancarlo, the noted restaurateur, succeeded in reversing his own type 2 diabetes using these recipes!

Omelettes Are Easy

···

Makes 1 omelette

Per serving: Total carbs 1 g, fibre 0 g, protein 17 g, fat 25 g, 296 kcal

On the surface, there's nothing simpler than making an omelette, right? But there are three things that will influence the outcome, and in order of importance they are:

1. The size of your frying pan: an overloaded pan will result in a spongy, undercooked eggy stodge; too big and you will end up with a thin, dry, almost inedible crisp.

2. Over-whisked eggs: a gentle swirl with a fork is all that is needed; no handheld or electric whisks please.

3. The choice of eggs: Burford Browns with their deep golden yolks are ideal, but any free-range variety will suffice.

Ingredients

- 3 medium free-range eggs
- a good knob of unsalted butter (approximately 15 g; you can use good-quality virgin olive oil in place of butter)
- salt and freshly ground black pepper

Method

1. Break the eggs into a bowl. Gently be until the yolks and whites combine, a add a generous whack of seasoning.

2. Warm a frying pan over a medium he Preferably, use a 26-cm (10-inch) pan for a three-egg omelette or a 21-cm (8-inch) pan for a two-egger.

3. Once the pan is hot, add the butter. (Waiting until the pan is hot means th butter won't overcook and brown.) Tu the heat right up and swirl the melted butter over the base and sides of the pan.

4. When the butter is frothing nicely, po in the eggs in one go and shake the pan vigorously so that everything is evenly spread out.

5. Now for the tricky bit. Using a fork or a small spatula, pull the edges of the omelette in from the sides of the par and, tipping the pan carefully, fill in t space left behind with the liquid egg that will be sitting in the middle. Kee doing this until the omelette is nearly set but the surface is still soft – know as *baveuse* in French, which means moist or a bit runny or undercooked. Don't forget the omelette will keep cooking while it's on your plate!

6. Holding the pan with one hand, tilt i over a plate and, with a fork, persuad the top edge to fold over the lower l before the omelette satisfyingly flop onto the plate.

ariations

ow you've mastered the omelette
aker's skill, you can add a range of
gredients to the egg mix – from
erbs to berries, and from cheese
vegetables and cooked meats.
ere are a few suggestions:

ne herbs

Add one level tablespoon of finely
chopped fresh parsley, chervil or chives
into the whisked eggs and stand in the
fridge for half an hour so the flavours
are established. Note: dried herbs just
don't cut it and can add an unpleasant
texture in the mouth.

Cook as per the instructions above.

Spinach, sun-dried tomato and goat's cheese

This appeared in *The Low-Carb Diabetes Cookbook* that Emma Porter and I published in 2018. This particular version is brilliant eaten cold out of the fridge in place of a sandwich.

1. Drain three sun-dried tomatoes of their oil and chop into small bite-sized pieces.

2. When the butter starts to froth, add the chopped tomatoes and stir for 60 seconds.

3. Add a handful of washed spinach leaves and wilt for another 60 seconds before pouring in the egg mixture.

4. As the omelette starts to firm up, dot it with a few pieces of chopped goat's cheese.

5. Once folded and on the plate, sprinkle with some fresh chives.

Other ingredients that work well in omelettes

+ Ham.

+ Sliced ripe tomatoes: grill the slices first until the edges are black and add as the omelette begins to set.

+ Sliced mushrooms: precook in a separate pan.

+ Sliced chorizo: precook in a separate pan.

+ Grated cheese, especially mature Cheddar, Parmesan and crumbled feta. Knobs of goat's cheese and soft blue cheeses can be added late in the cooking process.

+ Onions and leeks: precook in the pan before adding the eggs.

+ Grilled aubergine slices or thinly sliced avocado: can be treated as a 'filling' as the omelette is folded.

Open-Faced Omelette

Serves 6 portions

Per serving: Total carbs 10 g, fibre 2 g, protein 25 g, fat 37 g, 465 kcal

Travelling south from France, one encounters a quite different sort of omelette and if the folded version can be thought of as a sandwich substitute, then its open-faced cousin is more adjacent to a pizza. It keeps brilliantly in the fridge and can be served cold the next day.

Ingredients

- 1 (250 g, 8½ oz) courgette, trimmed and cut into ½-cm (¼-inch) rounds
- 2 tbsp plain flour, for dusting the courgettes
- 4 tbsp extra-virgin olive oil
- 6 large free-range eggs
- 50 g (1¾ oz) mature Cheddar cheese, finely grated
- 1 large Spanish onion, roughly chopped
- 1 fat garlic clove, peeled, finely chopped and crushed with the back of a knife
- 100 g (3½ oz) frozen peas
- 1 red pepper, deseeded and chopped into 1-cm (½-inch) pieces
- a handful of flat-leaf parsley, washed and finely chopped
- 200 g (7 oz) chorizo, skin removed and roughly chopped
- salt and freshly ground black pepper

Method

1. Place the rounds of courgette on a plate lined with kitchen paper, without overlapping. Sprinkle generously with salt, cover with more kitchen paper and place a second plate upside down on top with a saucepan to act as a press. Leave to drain for around 30 minutes.

2. Wash and pat dry the courgette before lightly sprinkling with flour. Heat three tablespoons of the oil in a frying pan over a medium heat and cook the courgettes for around 8 minutes. Set aside.

3. In a large bowl, gently whisk the eggs and combine with the grated cheese. Season with salt and plenty of black pepper. Set aside.

4. Heat the remaining oil in the frying pan over a moderate heat. Add the onion and sauté for around 5 minutes until soft, before adding the garlic. Cook for around 3 minutes, stirring continuously and then add the peas, red pepper and cooked courgettes. Cook for another 3 minutes or so.

5. Pour in the egg and cheese mixture along with the parsley and the chopped chorizo. Mix well and cook on a low heat for around 8–10 minutes.

6. Preheat the grill to high and finish the omelette under the grill for around 5 minutes.

7. Serve in individual wedges with a leaf salad.

Simple Stock

....

Makes 1 litre

arlier I urged you to replace the
nchtime sandwich with a bowl of
up, but it's worth noting that many
ands of tinned soup can contain
gnificant amounts of added sugar.
eally, and if time permits, make your
wn. The secret of a good soup will
e in the quality of the underlying
ock, so you will need to choose
etween using store-bought stocks
ubes, pots and 500-g packs) or
aking your own. The latter will
ways add a noticeable depth of
vour, but there is nothing wrong
th using the shop-bought variety.

eat stocks can take a while
d are something I dedicate
Saturday morning to. Making
gger batches for the freezer
o makes economic sense.

se ingredients

2 onions, chopped into quarters

2 celery sticks, roughly chopped

2 carrots, peeled and roughly
chopped

a handful of fresh parsley and thyme

1 bay leaf

1 litre (2 pints) cold water

a small palmful of black and white
peppercorns

For brown stock

Brown stock makes great gravies,
sauces and richly flavoured soups.

Method

1. Preheat the oven to 200°C (400°F, gas
   mark 6).

2. Spread 1½ kg (3⅓ lb) of raw beef, lamb
   or game bones plus any trimmings
   in a large roasting tin. Tuck in the
   vegetables and roast in the oven for 45
   minutes, or until everything has turned
   dark but not black.

3. Tip into a saucepan with the aromatics
   and cover with cold water.

4. Boil, then simmer over a very low heat
   with a tightly fitted lid for 4–8 hours
   for red meat bones, or 2–4 hours for
   poultry.

For white stock

This dispenses with the browning
step and results in a paler colour
and altogether gentler flavour.

Method

1. Put the raw bones or carcass,
   vegetables and aromatics straight into
   a saucepan and cover with cold water.
   Simmer for 1½–2 hours.

For fish stock

Method

1. Put approximately 500 g (17¾ oz) of the bones and trimmings from white fish, or alternatively shellfish shells, into a saucepan with the vegetables and aromatics, and cover with cold water.

2. Simmer for 30 minutes at the most.

For vegetable stock

Method

1. Put the vegetables and aromatics in a saucepan and cover with cold water. By all means include a trimmed leek and a few mushrooms that are about to give up the ghost.

2. Simmer for 30–45 minutes.

For all stocks

Method

1. A clear and pleasant tasting stock magically arises from a slow, gentle simmer. You will see a white froth rise to the surface. Using a large spoon, remove as much of it as you can. You will probably need to do this at least three or four times.

2. Once the stock has reached boiling point and you have skimmed and skimmed again, reduce the heat until you have only the faintest hint of bubbles rising to the surface. Put the lid on and leave well alone (other than checking the water level hasn't dropped too much – you can always top it up with boiling water).

3. Once the stock is ready, use a slotted spoon to remove the vegetables, bones, etc. and pass it through a fine sieve (or a muslin if you want a very refined stock). Allow it to cool completely before scooping away any final layer of surface fat.

The cooled stock will keep in the fridge for 3 days and in the freezer for several months.

Curried Parsnip Soup

·· ·· ·· ·· ·· ·· ·· ·· ·· ·· ·· ·· ·· ·· ·· ·· ·· ·· ·· ··

Serves 4 portions

Per serving: Total carbs 15 g, fibre 4 g, protein 2 g, fat 5 g, 70 kcal

delicious winter warmer that with
moderate use of chilli allows the
atural flavour of the vegetables
shine through. You can swap the
arsnips for carrots if you like.

gredients

1 tsp coriander seeds*

1 tsp cumin seeds*

1 tsp black peppercorns*

½ tsp turmeric*

½ tsp Kashmiri chilli powder*

2 garlic cloves, peeled

1 × 2-cm (1-inch) piece of root ginger,
peeled and roughly chopped

2 medium (or 1 large) white onions

3 tbsp extra-virgin olive oil

2 parsnips (or carrots), peeled and
roughly chopped

1½ litres (2½ pints) chicken or
vegetable stock or water

2 tsp garam masala

a bunch of fresh coriander, washed
and chopped

salt, to taste

1 tbsp full-fat Greek-style yoghurt,
to serve

* use Spice Mountain's Pav Bhaji
egetarian curry) mix

Method

1. If you are making your own spice mix,
place the coriander seeds, cumin
seeds and black peppercorns in a dry,
heavy-bottomed frying pan and heat
until they start to emit their natural oils,
about 3–4 minutes. Transfer to a spice
grinder and grind to a fine powder.
Alternatively, you can use a pestle and
mortar but it's hard work. Now add
the turmeric and chilli powder and set
aside.

2. Put the garlic, ginger and half of one of
the onions (or a quarter of a large onion
if using) along with one tablespoon
of water into a small blender and blitz
until you have a smooth paste. Add
the spice mix and blitz again until
everything is thoroughly mixed. It will
smell divine.

3. Roughly chop the remaining onions.
Add the oil to a deep, heavy-bottomed
saucepan and gently heat. Add the
remaining onions and stir until they
start to soften, around 4–5 minutes.
Ensure the onions are evenly spread
on the base of the saucepan and leave
on a gentle heat for another 5 minutes
or so without stirring until they are just
starting to brown.

4. Add the onion and spice mixture and
give everything a good stir. It will smell
even more wonderful. Keep stirring so
nothing catches. After a few minutes
add the parsnips, making sure they are
well coated.

5. Add the stock or water and bring to a very gentle simmer. Fit a tight lid and cook for around 30 minutes on a very low heat.

6. Add the garam masala and half the coriander and cook for a further 15 minutes.

7. Remove from the heat and allow to cool before blitzing with either a handheld or a kitchen-top blender. Once you have a really smooth consistency, adjust the seasoning.

8. To serve, dollop a large dessertspoonful of full-fat Greek-style yoghurt in the middle of each bowlful and sprinkle with the remaining coriander.

Carrot and Coriander Soup

Serves 4–6 portions

Per serving: Total carbs 6 g, fibre 1.6 g, protein 1 g, fat 10 g, 110 kcal

arrot soup (Potage de Crécy) is a
sh that has a status as a 'classic'
French cuisine and is named after
récy-en-Ponthieu, a commune
Northern France that allegedly
oduces the best-flavoured carrots
the country. Traditionally, Potage
Crécy includes potato and rice.
stead you can thicken the soup
th a good slosh of double cream.

gredients

2 tbsp extra-virgin olive oil

1 tsp ground black peppercorns

1 white onion, roughly chopped

800 g (25 oz) carrots, peeled and
roughly chopped

2 celery sticks, finely chopped

30 g (1 oz) fresh coriander

1½ litres (2½ pints) vegetable (or
chicken) stock, home-made or shop-
bought

salt, to taste

2 tbsp double cream, to serve
(optional)

Method

1. Pour the oil into a deep, heavy-
   bottomed saucepan and gently heat.
   Add the ground peppercorns and stir
   until they sizzle and emit their natural
   oils, about 3–4 minutes.

2. Add the onions and stir as they begin
   to soften. Leave without stirring (to
   caramelise) for 5 minutes until they are
   translucent and on the edge of turning
   brown.

3. Now add the carrots and celery. Give
   everything a good stir, turn up the heat
   and brown the vegetables for around
   5–6 minutes.

4. Meanwhile, chop the stalks from the
   coriander leaves and chuck them into
   the browning vegetable mix, reserving
   the leaves for later.

5. Pour in the stock, fit a tight lid and cook
   on a low heat for around 30 minutes, or
   until the vegetables are properly soft.

6. Remove from the heat and add the
   coriander leaves. Give everything a
   good stir and allow to cool before
   blitzing to a nice smooth texture.

7. Season with salt to taste and serve with
   a generous splash of cream (if using).

Chicken and Chard Soup

Serves 6 portions

Per serving: Total carbs 23.6 g, fibre 5.9 g, protein 28.3 g, fat 10 g, 308 kcal

Archaeological evidence shows that people started using poultry to make soups soon after they discovered how to boil water, and chicken soup has long been regarded as a therapeutic dish in several cultures. The second-century Greek physician Galen recommended chicken soup as a cure for migraine, leprosy, constipation and fever. Modern science has demonstrated that a bowl of chicken soup can have a mild anti-inflammatory effect and it is also said to be calming, which has led some to claim that it can also heal the soul. In short, everyone should have a chicken soup recipe in their repertoire!

Ingredients

- 2 tbsp virgin olive oil
- 200 g (7 oz) Swiss chard, washed and stems chopped
- 1 large onion, finely sliced into half moons
- 2 carrots, peeled and grated
- 1 × 400-g (14-oz) can chopped tomatoes
- 2 tsp fresh rosemary leaves, washed and chopped
- 1 tsp chilli flakes (optional, or add an extra tsp if you like the added heat)
- 1 litre (2 pints) chicken stock
- 1 × 400-g (14-oz) can red kidney beans, washed under running water in a sieve
- 2 roast chicken breasts*, meat shredded
- 2 tbsp Parmesan cheese, grated, plu extra for serving
- salt and freshly ground black peppe to taste

Method

1. Pour the oil into a deep, heavy-bottomed saucepan and gently heat. Add the chard stems, onions and carrot and sauté while gently stirring for 5 minutes before adding the charc leaves. Sauté for another 2 minutes or until the leaves have wilted.

2. Add the tomatoes , rosemary leaves and chilli flakes (if using) and give everything a good stir. Now add the stock and bring to a gentle boil.

3. Reduce the heat to low, add the bean cover and cook for 10 minutes.

4. Stir in the chicken and simmer for another 10 minutes.

5. Finally, stir in the grated Parmesan an season to taste.

6. Serve with extra cheese if you like.

* To roast chicken breasts: 1. Pat dry. 2. Place on a lightly oiled baking tray, sme with olive oil, season and bake in a pre-heated oven at 180°C for 25-30 minutes.

Pizza al Taglio (by the slice)

· ·

Serves 6 portions

Per serving: Total carbs 3.5 g, fibre 6.8 g, protein 21 g, fat 33 g, 409 kcal

This light, airy dough is easier and quicker to make than traditional wheat dough. There is no rising time, and the base contains a fraction of the carbs of a traditional pizza. Avoid buying ready-grated mozzarella as some brands contain potato starch, upping the carb content. Brown flaxseed is fine to use, but the pizza base will appear darker.

Ingredients

For the base

extra-virgin olive oil, to grease, plus extra for drizzling

75 g (2¾ oz) golden flaxseed, ground in a food processor to a sand-like texture

100 g (3½ oz) ground almonds

1 tsp baking powder

1 tsp salt

3 medium free-range eggs, lightly beaten

50 ml (2 fl oz) mozzarella brine from the bag, or water

For the tomato sauce

½ × 400-g (14-oz) can chopped tomatoes

1 tsp dried oregano

½ tsp salt

1 tbsp extra-virgin olive oil

To serve

- a handful of basil and rocket leaves (optional)
- 2 slices of prosciutto (optional)

Topping ideas

+ 12 black or green pitted olives, halved

+ 12 slices of salami or ham

+ 12 onion rings

+ dabs of a creamy blue cheese or goat's cheese

+ 25 g (1 oz) mushrooms, sliced

+ chilli flakes (to taste)

+ 1 × 110-g (3¾-oz) can tuna

+ 1 × 125-g (4½-oz) ball of mozzarella, finely chopped or grated

Method

1. Preheat the oven to 200°C (400°F, gas mark 6). Line a 35 × 25-cm (14 × 10-inch) baking tray with baking parchment and lightly brush with oil.

2. To make the pizza base, mix the dry ingredients together in a large mixing bowl with a metal spoon. Stir in the eggs and mozzarella brine or water. When you have a well-combined dough, relax for 10 minutes and let the dough do the same. The flaxseed will absorb the water. Use your hands to gather the dough into a ball.

3. Put the dough onto the prepared tray and press and shape it with wet hands

so that it fills the tray to a depth of just less than 1 cm (½ inch). Score with a knife into 6 or 12 divisions and bake for 8 minutes or until it feels firm to the touch. Do not let it brown.

4. While the base is in the oven, make the sauce by blending the ingredients together with a handheld blender in a bowl until smooth.

5. Take the base out of the oven and increase the temperature to 220°C (425°F, gas mark 7). Loosen the pizza from the tray (to check it will lift off eventually, but leave it in place on the tray) and make sure the score lines are visible. If not, go over them again.

6. Top the divisions with the tomato sauce or leave some without. Add your chosen topping(s) and dab on some additional mozzarella. Drizzle everything with a little extra-virgin oliv oil.

7. Bake for 8 minutes or until the mozzarella is bubbling and the crust is browned and nice and crisp. Remove from the oven and top with basil, rock and prosciutto, if using.

This recipe is taken from *The Reverse Your Diabetes Cookbook: Lose Weight and Eat to Beat Type 2 Diabetes* by Katie and Giancarlo Caldesi, published by Kyle Books (2020).

A Basic Curry Sauce

·····································

Makes enough for use in 8 2-person dishes

is said that the most closely
arded secret of any Indian
staurant is their recipe for a base
rry sauce. However much individual
efs claim that theirs is the best, the
sics will always be the same and
s home-made version can act as a
undation for almost any curry dish
egetarian or meat-based. It stores
ll in the freezer and will significantly
t down the time needed to prepare
imple curry dish and help you
oid the siren call of the takeaway.

e following dishes can all be served
h the Kachumber Salad on page
2 in place of rice or naan bread.

gredients

5 garlic cloves, peeled

2 x 2-cm (1-inch) piece of root ginger,
peeled and roughly chopped

6 medium onions

1½ litres (2½ pints) cold water

1 level tsp salt

1 x 400-g (14-oz) can chopped
tomatoes

a good glug of virgin olive oil

1 heaped tsp tomato puree

1 tsp turmeric

1½ tsp paprika

Method

1. Put the garlic cloves, chopped ginger and half of one of the onions along with a couple of teaspoons of water in a small blender and blitz until you have a smooth paste.

2. Roughly chop the remaining onions and place in a deep, heavy-bottomed saucepan and cover with the water. Stir in the garlic and ginger paste. Add the salt and gently bring to the boil. Turn down the heat, fit a tight lid and simmer for around 45 minutes.

3. Remove from the heat and allow to cool before blitzing in a blender to the smoothest consistency you can achieve. Wash out the saucepan and pour the blitzed onions back into it.

4. Wash out your blender and then blitz the canned tomatoes. Again, blitz to the smoothest consistency possible.

5. In a deep, non-stick or heavy-bottomed frying pan, pour in the oil and bring up to a moderate heat. Add the tomato puree, turmeric and paprika, stirring all the time.

6. Give it a few minutes stirring all the time before adding the tomatoes. Cook on a medium heat (the tomatoes should just about bubble) for 10 minutes, stirring regularly.

7. Now tip and scrape the cooked tomato and spice mix into the onion mixture. Stir and bring to the boil once more.

8. You will see a sort of froth rise to the surface of the sauce. It is vital you skim this off with a spoon. Expect to have to do this several times.

9. Simmer for 25 minutes, stirring from time to time. You should have a reasonably thick, red-coloured sauce that can be used straight away, kept in the fridge for 3 days or frozen into 8 portions (for 2-person meals) or 4 portions for 4-person meals.

This recipe is taken from *The Reverse Your Diabetes Cookbook: Lose Weight and Eat to Beat Type 2 Diabetes* by Katie and Giancarlo Caldesi, published by Kyle Books (2020).

Lamb Pasanda

....

Serves 4 portions

Per serving: Total carbs 15 g, fibre 4.5 g, protein 55 g, fat 78 g, 910 kcal

very family has someone who is
ot keen on spicy food and whose
eart sinks when the word 'curry' is
entioned. Well, this recipe is for
em. It is not at all spicy – in fact
is positively creamy, and if that
oesn't convince, you should add
at the dish was originally served
 Mughal emperors. The word
asanda' translates from Urdu
 'favourite', and refers to the
pensive cut of meat that was used.

gredients

450 g (1 lb) leg of lamb, diced into
bite-sized pieces

1 tbsp salt

200 ml (6¾ fl oz) full-fat plain Greek-
style yoghurt

4 tbsp extra-virgin olive oil

425 ml (15 fl oz) curry sauce

1 tsp paprika

1 tsp ground cumin

1 tsp garam masala

a handful of roughly chopped
almonds

4 tbsp double cream

1 tbsp fresh coriander, finely chopped

Method

1. Cover the lamb in cold water in a
   saucepan, add one teaspoon of the salt
   and gently bring to the boil. Cover and
   allow to simmer for around 30 minutes
   or until the meat is tender.

2. Mix the yoghurt with a further teaspoon
   of the salt in a bowl and add the meat
   while it is still warm. Allow the meat
   to marinate for at least 2 hours or
   overnight in the fridge once it's cooled.

3. Heat the oil in a deep, heavy-bottomed
   frying pan, add the curry sauce, paprika
   and the remaining salt. Allow the sauce
   to boil and simmer vigorously for 5
   minutes, stirring all the time.

4. Reduce the heat and stir in the cumin,
   garam masala and the almonds, and
   cook through for 3 minutes.

5. Remove the lamb from the yoghurt
   marinade and add to the frying pan.
   Cook for another 5 minutes or so.

6. Skim off any excess oil that's risen to
   the surface and stir in the cream and
   half of the coriander. Simmer for 4–5
   minutes.

7. Sprinkle the remaining coriander on
   top of each serving.

Paneer Tikka

....

Makes 6 skewers

Per serving: Total carbs 6 g, fibre 1 g, protein 15.5 g, fat 33 g, 233 kcal

I am grateful to the wonderful folk at Borough Market's Spice Mountain (www.spicemountain.co.uk) for this lovely veggie alternative for tandoori cooking made with paneer. Paneer is an Indian cheese that is firm and very mild, and which will soften but not melt when it is cooked. Because it has a neutral flavour, it will take on the smoky, spicy flavours of the marinade brilliantly. You will need at least six metal BBQ skewers for this recipe.

Ingredients

- 500 g (17½ oz) paneer cut into 2-cm (1-inch) cubes
- 1 large green pepper, deseeded and diced into 2-cm (1-inch) cubes
- 1 onion, diced into 2-cm (1-inch) cubes

For the marinade

- 2 tbsp mustard oil
- 2 tsp ginger garlic paste
- 250 ml (8½ oz) Greek yoghurt
- 3 tsp tandoori marinade
- 1 tsp chaat masala
- ½ tsp garam masala
- 2 tsp methi (fenugreek) leaves
- 1 tbsp lemon or lime juice

To serve and garnish

- ½ red onion, thinly sliced
- small handful of fresh coriander, chopped
- 1 lemon and/or lime, cut into wedg

Method

1. Mix together all the ingredients for th marinade and add the paneer cubes, coating them well. Allow the paneer marinate for at least 2 hours, preferab longer, in the fridge.

2. When you are ready to cook, prehea the oven to 220°C (425°F, gas mark 7 then set about alternatively skewerin the marinated paneer with the green pepper and onion.

3. Position the skewers on a rack and bake for 15 minutes, turning halfway through. To get the paneer charred, either move them to the top of the oven for a little while or finish them off under a high grill (or you can use cook's blowtorch which is always fun!

4. Place the skewers carefully onto a serving platter and garnish with the onion and coriander. Sit some lemor and/or lime wedges on the plate to squeeze over.

Vegetable Sambar

···

Serves 4 portions

Per serving: Total carbs 26 g, fibre 8.4 g, protein 14.5 g, fat 16.1, 346 kcal

ırry leaves, plenty of black pepper,
illi for heat and tamarind for
urness are the hallmarks of South
dian cookery and this sambar
akes a wonderful light meal. By all
eans use fresh curry leaves if you
n find them, but dried ones work
rfectly well for this soup-like recipe.

gredients

150 g (5½ oz) split yellow lentils

3 tbsp cold-pressed rapeseed oil

3 whole Kashmiri chillies, plus 2 to
serve

2 tsp coriander seeds

½ tsp fenugreek seeds

1½ tsp cumin seeds

2 tbsp desiccated coconut

2 tsp mustard seeds

2 tsp ground black peppercorns

4 shallots, finely chopped

10 dried curry leaves

450 g (16 oz) vegetables, such as
carrots, butternut squash, aubergine
and green beans, all cut into bite-
sized pieces

3 medium tomatoes, sliced

1½ tsp salt

1½ tsp tamarind paste

Method

1. Put the lentils into a small colander and wash thoroughly under cold running water until the water runs clear.

2. Tip the lentils into a saucepan, cover with approximately three or four times the amount of water and bring to the boil. Simmer for around 40 minutes, regularly skimming off the foam that will rise to the surface. Be careful not to allow the lentils to dry out during the cooking period. You can always top up with boiling water. Once cooked, you should end up with a wet, soup-like consistency.

3. While the lentils (henceforth called the dal) are simmering, heat one tablespoon of the oil in a small, heavy-bottomed frying pan and add the chillies, and the coriander, fenugreek and cumin seeds. Stir-fry for 1 minute or until the coriander seeds start to turn golden, then add the coconut for just a minute. Allow to cool for a few minutes before grinding the spice mix to a paste in a grinder or a pestle and mortar.

4. Heat the remaining oil in a large frying pan on a medium heat and add the mustard seeds, which will jump about, the black pepper, the shallots and finally the curry leaves. Give everything a good stir. Sauté until the shallots have turned translucent and started to brown – around 10–15 minutes.

5. Start to add the vegetables, beginning with the carrots, squash and aubergine. Cover with a lid and cook for around 5 minutes before adding the beans and the tomatoes and a drop of water to loosen everything. Cover and leave to cook for a further 5 minutes.

6. Stir in the spice paste, salt and tamarind paste. Cover and cook for another 5 minutes.

7. Once you are happy that the vegetables and tomatoes are cooked, transfer everything into the dal, stir to mix and adjust the seasoning. Top with a couple of quickly oil-fried Kashmiri chillies and you're ready to serve.

Chicken Jalfrezi

....

Serves 4–6 portions

Per serving: Total carbs 28 g, fibre 4.5 g, protein 20 g, fat 35 g, 653 kcal

jalfrezi, along with the ubiquitous
icken tandoori, remains among the
ost popular of restaurant curries. It
as the invention of the Raj where it
as designed to use up leftovers by
ing them with onions and chilli. It
dry without lots of gravy and with
hick sauce that clings beautifully
the main ingredient. The flavour
ould be hot, sour and with a
te of sweetness from the lightly
oked onions and green pepper.
frezi can be made with any meat,
afood or vegetable, but a particular
ourite is paneer (Indian cheese).

gredients

½ tsp turmeric

1 × 2-cm (1-inch) piece of root ginger,
peeled and grated

1 tbsp garam masala

1 tbsp amchur (dried green mango
powder)

a pinch of salt

1 tsp Kashmiri chilli powder

1 tbsp ground cumin

4 tbsp cold-pressed rapeseed oil

4 boneless, skinless chicken breasts,
dried on a paper towel and cut into
bite-sized pieces

1 medium onion, roughly quartered

- 1 green pepper, deseeded and cut into strips
- 1 × 210-g (7½-oz) can chopped tomatoes
- 3 long green chillies, deseeded and finely chopped, plus 2 cut lengthways to garnish
- 200 ml (6¾ fl oz) curry sauce
- 2 firm tomatoes, skin on and cut into wedges
- a handful of fresh coriander, chopped

Method

1. In a non-metallic bowl, mix the turmeric, ginger, garam masala, amchur, salt, chilli powder, cumin and one tablespoon of the oil. Add the chicken pieces and mix thoroughly. Cover with clingfilm and marinate in the fridge for 2–3 hours or overnight. Remember to bring it back to room temperature before cooking the chicken.

2. Heat one-and-a-half tablespoons of the oil in a large, deep, non-stick or heavy-bottomed frying pan (or a karahi, in which case you will need to have everything ready to go as you won't be able to take your eyes off it) over a high heat. Add the onions and pepper and sauté for 3–4 minutes. The onion should become translucent but must not brown.

3. Reduce the heat somewhat and add the chopped tomatoes and cook for

another couple of minutes. Transfer the contents of the pan to a bowl and set aside.

4. Return the pan to the heat and add the remaining oil. Once hot, stir in the well-shaken chicken pieces and sauté for around 5 minutes, turning them over from time to time. Add the chopped chillies and sauté for another minute or so.

5. Now add the curry sauce to the pan and cook until much of the liquid has evaporated and the chicken is cooked – around 5–6 minutes.

6. Tip the bowl of fried vegetables into the chicken, stir and cook for another minutes.

7. Add the tomato wedges and cook for 2–3 minutes more and, finally, add the halved chillies. Sprinkle with coriander and serve. Depending on the strength of the chillies, it's worth having a pot of yoghurt or a raita standing by.

Sri Lankan Vegetable and Coconut Curry

Serves 4 portions

Per serving: Total carbs 22 g, fibre 10 g, protein 9.8 g, fat 43 g, 532 kcal

is terrific curry recipe is supplied Katie Caldesi, author of several stselling low-carb recipe books.

gredients

1 tsp coriander seeds

1 tsp cumin seeds

2-cm (1-inch) cinnamon stick

½ tsp turmeric

3 cardamom pods, husks discarded

1 tsp fenugreek seeds

15 curry leaves, fresh or dried

2 tbsp extra-virgin olive oil

1 × 2-cm (1-inch) piece of root ginger, peeled and finely chopped

2 fat garlic cloves, peeled and finely chopped

2 green chillies, split in half

1 leek, approx. 200 g (7 oz), trimmed and roughly chopped

500 g (17 oz) low-carb vegetables, such as green beans, cauliflower, mushrooms and courgette, cut into bite-sized pieces

1 × 400-g (14-oz) can chickpeas, drained

2 × 400-g (14-oz) cans coconut milk

salt and freshly ground black pepper, to taste

Method

1. Toast all the spices in a dry frying pan for a minute or two until they release their aroma; pick out the cinnamon stick and set aside and then grind the rest to a fine powder in a spice grinder or pestle and mortar. Don't worry if the curry leaves don't break down completely.

2. Heat the oil in a deep, heavy-bottomed saucepan or frying pan over a medium heat and stir in the powdered spices, cinnamon stick, ginger, garlic and chillies. Cook for a couple of minutes, stirring constantly with a wooden spoon.

3. Add the leek and other vegetables, chickpeas, coconut milk and seasoning. Bring to the boil, then reduce the heat and cook for around 10 minutes or until just tender, stirring frequently and pushing the vegetables under the surface of the liquid as much as you can.

4. Taste and adjust the seasoning if necessary. Remove the chillies. Spoon the curry into warm bowls and eat straight away or cool and keep for up to 3 days in the fridge. This is ideal for taking to work warm in a thermos flask or reheating at work in a microwave.

Kachumber Salad

· ·

Serves 4 portions

Per serving: Total carbs 8 g, fibre 3 g, protein 1 g, fat 0 g, 45 kcal

This tangy, colourful Indian cucumber salad is delicious served with a curry. It's a simple fresh salad with sliced onions, tomatoes, cucumber and a lemon (or lime) juice dressing. You can always add mint leaves and a splash of yoghurt.

Ingredients

- 1 red onion, finely sliced into half moons
- 1 large cucumber, washed, topped and tailed, cut in half vertically and diced
- 300 g (10½ oz) cherry tomatoes, cut in half (depending on size)
- 1 green chilli, deseeded and finely chopped
- 1 large carrot, peeled and grated or julienned
- 5 medium radishes, finely sliced
- ½ tsp rock salt (or to taste)
- ½ tsp ground black pepper
- ½ tsp ground cumin
- ½ tsp Kashmiri chilli powder (optional)
- 2 tbsp fresh lemon or lime juice

Method

1. Prepare the vegetables and toss in a large bowl with the seasoning and spices. Pour over the lemon or lime juice. Simples.

A Simple Chinese-Style Stir-Fry

Serves 2 portions

Per serving: Total carbs 9 g, fibre 5 g, protein 3 g, fat 14 g, 210 kcal

ᴜ can usually find pre-packed
ᴠegetables trimmed and prepared for
-frying in supermarkets and they
ke for a quick and tasty evening
al or as an accompaniment to any
ᴉnese-influenced dish, such as the
ast Salmon with Sesame and Spring
ᴉon Crust (page 348). All you need is
ᴦge wok of reasonable quality and a
ᴉple of oils and you're ready to go.

ᵧredients

1 tbsp sesame seeds

2 tbsp groundnut oil

1 medium onion, roughly chopped

¼ green chilli, deseeded and finely
sliced on the diagonal

1 × 300-g (10½-oz) pack stir-fry
vegetables that ideally includes
spring onions, ginger, bamboo shoots
and water chestnuts

1 tbsp Chinese rice wine (optional)

1 tbsp toasted sesame oil

salt and freshly ground black pepper,
to taste

tamari or soy sauce, to serve

Method

1. Put the sesame seeds in a hot, dry
   frying pan and fry until they adopt a
   warm golden colour (about 3 minutes).
   Turn out onto a plate and allow to cool.

2. Heat the groundnut oil in a wok (a large
   frying pan will suffice but somehow
   doesn't quite deliver the same result)
   over a high temperature until it's really
   hot, swirling the oil against the sides of
   the wok all the time.

3. Add the onions and chilli and stir-fry for
   2 minutes before adding the rest of the
   vegetables.

4. Stir-fry for another 3–4 minutes, stirring
   all the time, with the occasional toss
   if you've got the technique to match,
   until the vegetables are soft but still
   have a crunch. Stir in the Chinese rice
   wine (if using) and sesame oil. Season
   to taste and serve scattered with the
   toasted sesame seeds and plenty of
   tamari or soy sauce.

343

A Simple Village Salad

···

Serves 2 portions

Per serving: Total carbs 15.9 g, fibre 5.5 g, protein 17.3 g, fat 38 g, 482 kcal

Katie Caldesi discovered this simple salad on a trip to Cyprus. It will go well with just about any of the dishes presented here.

Ingredients

- 1 small red onion, finely sliced
- ½ long cucumber, cubed
- 1 green pepper, deseeded and cut into bite-sized pieces
- 2 large ripe tomatoes, top cores removed, roughly chopped
- 10 Kalamata olives, stoned
- 2 tbsp extra-virgin olive oil
- 1 tbsp red wine vinegar
- a small bunch of flat-leaf parsley, leaves roughly chopped and stalks finely chopped
- 200 g (7 oz) feta cheese
- salt and freshly ground black pepper, to taste

Method

1. Combine all the ingredients, apart from the cheese, in a mixing bowl and season to taste.
2. Divide between two bowls and coarse grate the cheese over the top. Serve straight away or leave in the fridge for up to an hour.

Ricotta Pancakes with Cinnamon Apples and Whipped Cream

....

Serves 4 portions

Per serving: Total carbs 18 g, fibre 4.8 g, protein 25 g, fat 59 g, 680 kcal

ese light pancakes are great brunch. Cooked apples act a prebiotic, helping to feed good bacteria in your gut.

gredients

3 medium apples

25 g (1 oz) salted butter

1 tsp ground cinnamon

4 medium free-range eggs, with the yolks separated from the whites

150 g (5 oz) ricotta cheese

50 g (2 oz) ground almonds

1 tsp baking powder

1 tbsp extra-virgin olive oil

erve

150 ml (5 fl oz) double cream

2 tsp vanilla extract

50 g (1¾ oz) pecans, roughly chopped

thod

Whip the cream and vanilla extract ogether in a bowl until they form soft peaks. Keep chilled in the fridge until erving.

lice the apples into quarters leaving he skin on and remove the core from ach part. Cut each quarter into four ices.

3. Warm three-quarters of the butter and two tablespoons of water in a non-stick frying pan and, when bubbling, add the apple slices. Let them brown on one side and then flip over with a spatula. Scatter over the cinnamon and continue to cook for 7–10 minutes or until soft. Keep warm until needed.

4. Meanwhile, put the egg yolks, ricotta and dry ingredients into a large mixing bowl and mix thoroughly. In another bowl whisk the egg whites to stiff peaks and, using a large spoon, gently fold them into the egg yolk mixture.

5. Heat the oil and remaining butter in a non-stick frying pan. Drop two tablespoons of the mixture into the hot pan to make each pancake and flatten gently. You should be able to fit three or four in at one time. When they are risen and puffy, set underneath and lightly browned, flip to the other side with a spatula. Repeat with the remaining mixture using a little more oil as needed.

6. Serve the pancakes on individual plates dressed with the apples and any cooking juices from the pan, the cream and the pecans.

La Parmigiana di Melanzane (Aubergine Parmesan)

Serves 8 portions

Per serving: Total carbs 18 g, fibre 4.4 g, protein 44 g, fat 32 g, 482 kcal

A version of this recipe appeared in my earlier book *Reverse Your Diabetes: Diet* and I make no apologies for including it here. In the years that have passed since, I have refined the recipe somewhat and it has become my most requested dish. It is rustic, brilliant for sharing and ideally served with a large bowl of green salad and a glass or two of robust red wine. *Buon appetito!*

Ingredients

- 3 large aubergines, sliced into ¾-cm (⅓-in) roundels
- plenty of salt (don't worry, it will be washed off before cooking)
- 3 or 4 large free-range eggs
- 30 g (1 oz) plain flour, for dusting the aubergines slices
- 4 tbsp olive oil, or enough to completely cover the bottom of the pan to the depth of a few millimetres
- 2 × 125-g (4½-oz) packs mozzarella cheese, chopped into bite-sized pieces
- 2 × 60-g (2-oz) packs grated Parmigiano Reggiano cheese (or any good-quality Parmesan cheese – you can always do the grating yourself)

For the tomato sauce

- 60 ml (2 fl oz) extra-virgin olive oil
- freshly ground black pepper
- 1 tbsp tomato puree
- 2 large garlic cloves, peeled, finely chopped and lightly crushed with t back of a knife
- 2 glasses (100 ml / 3½ fl oz) of red wine (optional, but it makes a difference!)
- 2 × 400-g (14-oz) cans chopped tomatoes
- some overripe fresh tomatoes, skinned and chopped (optional)
- ⅔ × 500-g pack passata (smooth, thick, sieved tomatoes)
- salt
- a good handful of fresh basil leave torn (or 1 heaped tsp dried basil)

Method

1. To start, place the rounds of aubergi on a plate lined with kitchen paper, without overlapping. Sprinkle generously with salt, cover with anot piece of kitchen paper and repeat until all the aubergine is piled up wit interleaved kitchen paper. Place a second plate upside down on top. A a couple of saucepans to act as a 'pr and leave to drain for an hour or so.

Now, make the tomato sauce. Pour the extra-virgin olive oil into a large, heavy-bottomed saucepan and heat gently. Add the freshly ground pepper and tomato puree and allow to cook very gently with the occasional stir for 5 minutes.

Add the garlic and cook for no more than 3 minutes, ensuring it does not go beyond a very light gold colour.

Add the red wine (if using), turn up the heat and allow it to reduce down to almost nothing.

Add the canned tomatoes, fresh tomatoes (if using) and the passata. Stir well and simmer uncovered for 10 minutes. Add a pinch of salt, cover and cook on a gentle heat for around 30 minutes.

Finally, add the basil, remove from the heat and allow to cool.

Break the eggs into a bowl and whisk gently.

Wash and pat dry the aubergine before lightly sprinkling with flour.

Preheat the oven to 190°C (375°F, gas mark 5).

Warm the olive oil in a large, non-stick or heavy-bottomed frying pan on a moderate heat. Now dip each floured aubergine piece in the egg and place in the heated frying pan. Turn up the heat. Fry each pan's worth until the aubergines take on a dark (almost burnt) colour on both sides. Remove, place on a plate lined with kitchen paper and repeat with the next batch. The aubergines will soak up a lot of oil and this is a time- and labour-intensive process that can't be rushed, but it's well worth it.

11. To assemble the dish, spoon a layer of the tomato sauce on the bottom of an ovenproof dish (ideally a 23 x 33-cm / 9 x 13-inch lasagne dish), top with a layer of the aubergine and dot with mozzarella pieces. Spoon another layer of tomato sauce over the cheese before sprinkling with a generous helping of Parmesan. Start again with a new layer of aubergines and repeat until you have three layers of aubergine, tomato sauce, mozzarella and finally everything topped with Parmesan.

12. Bake in the oven for 35–45 minutes until the top is well browned but not black (if it starts to darken too much, cover with tin foil).

13. Allow to stand for 10 minutes before serving.

14. Once cooled, it can be stored in the fridge for 2–3 days and either eaten cold or reheated in the microwave.

Roast Salmon with Sesame and Spring Onion Crust

Serves 6 portions

Per serving: Total carbs 1.9 g, fibre 0 g, protein 40 g, fat 30 g, 438 kcal

This stunning salmon dish is easy to make, and the onion curls and sesame seeds can be prepared in advance. Serve with A Simple Chinese-Style Stir-Fry (page 342).

Ingredients

- 8 spring onions
- 2 tbsp sesame seeds
- 1 side of salmon (approximately 1 kg / 2lb 4 oz)
- 3 tbsp extra-virgin olive oil
- 1 tsp Szechuan or black peppercorns, crushed to a rough texture in a pestle and mortar
- 1 tsp toasted sesame oil
- 1 hot red chilli, peeled and finely sliced on the diagonal
- 2 fat garlic cloves, finely sliced
- 1 x 10-g (¼-oz) piece of root ginger, peeled and julienned (cut into fine strips)
- 2 tbsp tamari or soy sauce
- salt

Method

1. Preheat the oven to 200°C (400°F, gas mark 6).

2. Cut the green parts of the spring onions off and slice them into strips, keeping one end intact. Put them in a bowl of cold water to soak – they will curl. Cut the white parts diagonally a set aside.

3. Toast the sesame seeds in a dry pan until golden brown. Set aside.

4. Put the salmon in a roasting dish and brush with one tablespoon of the olive oil and season with salt and the crushed pepper. Roast for 20 minute or until firm to the touch and cooked through. Transfer to a serving plate a keep warm.

5. Heat the remaining olive oil and the sesame oil over a high heat and fry the chilli, the white part of the spring onions, the garlic and the ginger for 2–3 minutes until lightly golden in colour. Stir in the tamari or soy sauce and, as soon as it starts to bubble, p it over the salmon and dress with the toasted sesame seeds.

6. Finally, drain the green spring onion curls, separate them and scatter alongside or over the salmon and serve.

This recipe is taken from: *The Reverse Your Diabe* *Cookbook: Lose Weight and Eat to Beat Type 2 Diabetes* by Katie and Giancarlo Caldesi published by Kyle Books (2020).

Mushroom Cream Sauce with Leek 'Pasta'

Serves 2 portions

Per serving: Total carbs 16 g, fibre 2.5 g, protein 8.5 g, fat 11 g, 782 kcal

eaking the pasta habit of a lifetime
a challenge, but this luscious creamy
ashroom sauce served on a bed of
ks is as good a place to start as any.

gredients

1 heaped tsp black peppercorns

125 g (4½ oz) flat or Chestnut mushrooms, finely chopped

4 tbsp extra-virgin olive oil

½ small white onion or 1 banana shallot, finely chopped

2 garlic cloves, peeled and finely chopped

1 small glass (100 ml / 3½ fl oz) white wine

100 ml (3½ fl oz) double cream

50 g (1¾ oz) goat's cheese or a creamy blue cheese such as St Agur

½ tsp dried tarragon

2 medium (or 1 large) leeks, trimmed, washed and cut into ½-cm (¼-inch) roundels

a small knob of unsalted butter

salt

15–20 g (½–¾ oz) grated Parmesan, to serve

thod

Begin by crushing the black peppercorns to a reasonably fine texture in a pestle and mortar. (If you

like a little bit of chilli heat, you can add one very small dried red chilli or a few chilli flakes to the peppercorns.)

2. In a frying pan, sauté the chopped mushrooms in one tablespoon of the oil with a pinch of salt for around 5 minutes until they are well reduced and nicely browned. Set aside.

3. Put the remaining oil in a saucepan and gently heat before adding the crushed pepper. Let the pepper release its natural oils for a few minutes and then add the onion or shallot to the pan. Turn up the heat a fraction and cook until the onion is translucent – around 7 minutes.

4. Add the garlic and cook for just a few minutes – keep stirring so it doesn't darken and go bitter.

5. Add the wine and reduce to almost nothing.

6. Add the sautéed mushrooms to the pan along with the cream. Once it has warmed through enough to melt the cheese, add the cheese while stirring vigorously. Add the tarragon.

7. Allow to bubble very gently on the hob while you get on with the leeks. Adjust the seasoning, but, be careful, the Parmesan will add a salty note when you serve.

8. Using your thumb, push the tightly-packed interior of each leek roundel out and into a colander. Once you have done this with all the leeks, give them a good wash under running water

then put them in a largish frying pan with one tablespoon of water plus the butter. Fit a tight lid and cook on a medium heat for around 6 minutes or until the leeks are soft and cooked.

9. To serve, put the leeks into two bowls and spoon over the mushroom sauce Sprinkle generously with Parmesan. You will find the sweet taste of the lee complements the sauce perfectly.

Vegetarian Chilli (Non) Con Carne

....

Serves 6 portions

Per serving: Total carbs 19 g, fibre 7.4 g, protein 6.6 g, fat 5.1 g, 175 kcal

you prefer a meaty version, you
an add 450 g (15¾ oz) of browned
ince in place of the mushrooms
id carrots used here. You can
so adjust the amount of chilli,
it in my view this dish is best
rved hot and spicy, and reducing
e chilli turns it into something
uch more like a boring stew.

gredients

2 tbsp extra-virgin olive oil

1 tsp crushed black peppercorns

2 heaped tbsp tomato puree

2 medium (or 1 large) onions,
chopped

2 fat garlic cloves, peeled, finely
chopped and crushed with the back
of a knife

1 tsp Kashmiri chilli powder

1 tsp paprika

1 tsp cayenne pepper

4 large flat mushrooms, chopped
quite finely

1 × 400-g (14-oz) can chopped
tomatoes

570 ml (1 pint) vegetable stock (for
non-vegetarians, use chicken stock)

2 medium carrots, peeled and diced

1 green pepper, deseeded and
chopped

- 1 × 400-g (14-oz) can red kidney
  beans, washed under running water
  in a sieve
- salt, to taste

Method

1. Warm the oil in a large (28-cm or 11-
   in is ideal), deep, heavy-bottomed
   frying pan (or casserole dish). Add the
   peppercorns and the tomato puree.
   Spread everything about and allow
   to cook on a low heat for around 5
   minutes before adding the onions. Give
   it all a good stir to ensure everything is
   coated with the oil, pepper and puree
   mix, turn up the heat and allow to
   sweat until the onions have started to
   soften – around 6 minutes.

2. Add the garlic and stir. Now quickly
   add the chilli powder, paprika and
   cayenne pepper and cook while stirring
   for around 3 minutes.

3. Add the mushrooms and cook on a
   medium heat until they have largely
   reduced and a lot of their water content
   has evaporated.

4. Tip in the chopped tomatoes and cook
   for another 5 minutes while stirring.

5. Add the stock and the carrots, and give
   it a final stir. Fit a tight lid and simmer
   on the hob on a low to medium heat
   for around 30 minutes.

6. Remove the lid, add the green pepper and red kidney beans and cook until the stock has reduced so that you have a nearly dry chilli. This will take around 15 minutes.

7. Season with salt to taste and serve in individual bowls with a simple salad and a pot of plain, full-fat yoghurt. It keeps well in the fridge, and if anything tastes even better the next day.

Sausages with Roasted Vegetables

Serves 4 portions

Per serving: Total carbs 9.3 g, fibre 4.9 g, protein 25.9 g, fat 28.7 g, 409 kcal

nother Katie Caldesi recipe. Try
is easy traybake for a midweek
pper with beautiful Mediterranean
getables giving plenty of healthy
lour and variety. To keep the carbs
wn, look for sausages with a high
eat content rather than those filled
th rusk or flour. Have this on its
vn or with a crisp, green salad.

gredients

1 red Romano or bell pepper,
deseeded and cut into 8 strips

1 small onion, cut into 8 wedges

1 large courgette (200 g / 7 oz) or
4 baby courgettes, cut into 2-cm
(1-in) slices

300 g (10 oz) cauliflower or broccoli,
cut into bite-sized florets

3 tbsp extra-virgin olive oil

a handful of thyme sprigs or 2 tsp
dried thyme

8 sausages with a high meat content

salt and freshly ground black pepper

Method

1. Preheat the oven to 220°C (425°F, gas
   mark 7).

2. Toss the vegetables with the oil,
   seasoning and herbs in a large mixing
   bowl so that all the ingredients are
   coated.

3. Spread the mixture out into a
   single layer in a roasting tin or large
   ovenproof dish. Prick the skins of the
   sausages and tuck them between the
   vegetables.

4. Roast for 20–25 minutes, tossing the
   ingredients together once during the
   cooking time until the vegetables are
   golden brown and the sausages are
   cooked through.

Creamy Pork and Mushroom Stroganoff with Buttered Courgette Ribbons

Serves 4 portions

Per serving of pork stroganoff (excluding courgettes):
Total carbs 7.6 g, fibre 1.2 g, protein 31 g, fat 16 g, 320 kcal

Per serving of buttered courgettes:
Total carbs 1.4 g, fibre 2.7 g, protein 1.6 g, fat 17.8 g, 170 kcal

Katie says, 'I remember this classic dish from the 1980s as one of the recipes that my mother would cook when people came around. Giancarlo remembers creamy stroganoff being served with gherkins in restaurants in London when he came to the UK and worked as a waiter. Nowadays we eat it with the buttered courgette ribbons rather than rice or pasta.'

Ingredients

- 250 g (8¾ oz) chestnut mushrooms, sliced
- 1 medium white onion, finely chopped
- 2 garlic cloves, peeled and lightly crushed
- 4 tbsp extra-virgin olive oil
- 2 knobs of unsalted butter
- 500 g (1 lb) pork tenderloin, trimmed and cut into finger-sized strips
- 2 tsp unsmoked paprika or 1 flat tsp cayenne pepper
- 1 small glass (100 ml / 3½ fl oz) white wine
- 200 ml (6¾ fl oz) sour cream, doubl cream or full-fat crème fraîche
- 2 tsp Dijon mustard
- 1 tbsp lemon juice
- 65 g (2 oz) gherkins, finely choppec
- 300 g (10½ oz) courgettes, washed
- salt and freshly ground black peppe
- 2 tbsp roughly chopped parsley, to serve

Method

1. Fry the mushrooms, onions and garli with seasoning in two tablespoons of the oil and half a knob of butter in a frying pan over a medium heat for around 7–10 minutes. They are done when the water has evaporated from the mushrooms and the onions have softened.

2. Put the pork into a bowl with the paprika and a little seasoning. Toss through to coat it. Add the pork to the pan and stir through. Continue t fry for a few minutes then pour in the wine. Allow it to reduce for 5 minute before adding the sour cream, half a knob of butter, mustard, lemon juice and gherkins. Taste and adjust the seasoning as necessary.

. To make the buttered courgette ribbons, use a vegetable peeler to make long ribbons. Heat the remaining oil in a deep frying pan and add the courgette ribbons along with a pinch of salt and a crack of black pepper. Cook for around 8 minutes, stirring from time to time until the ribbons are soft but not soggy. Add a knob of butter and, once it melts, remove the pan from the heat and check the seasoning.

4. Pile the buttered courgette ribbons into warm bowls and put the pork stroganoff on the side. Scatter the pork with parsley and black pepper and serve straight away.

Quick and Spicy Chilli Beef

Serves 2 portions

Per serving: Total carbs 15 g, fibre 5.4 g, protein 48 g, fat 32 g, 556 kcal

You can make this delicious dish really quickly and in no time you have a substantial meal. Have on its own, with a dressed salad or baby spinach.

Ingredients

- 2 tbsp extra-virgin olive oil
- 1 red pepper, deseeded and thinly sliced
- 1 white onion, sliced into half moons
- 2 fat garlic cloves, peeled and crushed
- 300 g (10½ oz) minced beef with 15–20% fat
- ½ tsp hot chilli powder
- 1 tsp unsmoked sweet paprika
- ½ tsp ground cumin
- ½ tsp dried oregano
- ¼ tsp cinnamon powder
- 1 tbsp tomato puree
- 75 ml (2½ fl oz) cold water
- 100 g (3½ oz) cherry tomatoes, halved
- 125 g (4½ oz) mozzarella
- salt and freshly ground black pepper
- a small handful of coriander leaves, to serve

Method

1. Preheat the grill to hot.
2. Heat the oil in a large frying pan or wo and fry the pepper and onions over a high heat for around 5 minutes until they start to brown and soften. Add the garlic, minced beef, seasoning and spices and stir through. Cook for minutes until the beef is browned.
3. Mix the tomato puree with the water in a mug and add to the pan with the cherry tomatoes. Cook for 5 minutes until everything is piping hot. Taste ar adjust the seasoning to your liking.
4. Transfer to an ovenproof dish and tea the mozzarella over the top. Put on a high rack under the grill for 5–8 minut or until golden brown and bubbling and some of the meat has crispened. Remove from the grill and serve decorated with coriander leaves.

Calves' Liver with Butter and Sage

Serves 4 portions

Per serving: Total carbs 0.6 g, fibre 0 g, protein 28 g, fat 35 g, 410 kcal

his classic Italian dish makes a
outh-watering evening meal in
nly 3 minutes – the ultimate fast
od! And did you know that calves'
ver contains more vitamin C,
eight for weight, than an apple?
is a genuine superfood with more
utrients than most other foods and
something meat eaters should
clude more often in their diet.

gredients

4 pieces of calves' liver,
approximately 150 g (5½ oz) each

4 tbsp extra-virgin olive oil

4 garlic cloves, peeled and lightly
crushed with the back of a knife

75 g (2¼ oz) salted butter at room
temperature

8 large sage leaves

salt and freshly ground black pepper

Method

1. Season the liver on both sides.

2. Heat the oil in a large, non-stick frying
   pan over a medium heat, add the garlic
   and fry until it just starts to colour.

3. Turn up the heat to high and put the
   liver pieces into the pan. Fry for 30
   seconds on each side for medium
   cooked or 45 seconds for well done.

4. If your pan isn't big enough, fry the liver
   in two batches.

5. With the liver in the pan, reduce the
   heat, add the butter and sage leaves
   (halving quantity if cooking in two
   batches) to the pan and continue
   cooking the liver until the butter has
   melted.

6. Place each portion on a plate, pour
   over the butter and sage sauce and
   garlic and serve straight away. It goes
   well with sautéed spinach.

This recipe is taken from: *The Reverse Your Diabetes
Cookbook: Lose Weight and Eat to Beat Type 2
Diabetes* by Katie and Giancarlo Caldesi published
by Kyle Books (2020).

Scones with Strawberry Chia Jam

Makes 8 mini scones

Per scone: Total carbs 1.7 g, fibre 1.7 g, protein 4.1 g, fat 11 g, 126 kcal

These delightful little scones look pretty piled up on a cake stand. They are best cooked in mini-muffin moulds to maintain a good shape. Serve them with Strawberry Chia Jam and clotted or whipped cream. If you can find white chia seeds, the colour of the jam is brighter than if you use black seeds.

Ingredients

- 100 g (3½ oz) ground almonds
- 1 heaped tsp baking powder
- 30 g (1 oz) unsalted butter, melted
- 2 heaped tbsp natural yoghurt
- 1 tsp vanilla extract
- 1 large free-range egg

Method

1. To make the scones, preheat the oven to 180°C (350°F, gas mark 4).

2. Mix the dry ingredients together in a bowl. Add the butter, yoghurt and vanilla extract and stir through with a fork making sure they are well blended.

3. Separate the egg and put the egg white into a large bowl. Keep the yolk for the glaze. Whisk the white to form stiff peaks. Use a metal spoon to gently fold it into the almond mixture keeping as much air in as possible.

4. Divide the mixture between 8 silicone mini-muffin moulds or use mini-muffin cases. Using a pastry brush, glaze each mini-muffin with the egg yolk. Bake for 15 minutes or until golden and firm to the touch.

For the Strawberry Chia Jam

Serves 8 portions

Per serving of jam: Total carbs 6.4 g, fibre 5.1 g, protein 1.2 g, fat 1.5 g, 62 kcal

Ingredients

- 300 g (10½ oz) strawberries, hulled and roughly chopped
- 1 tbsp chia seeds
- 1 tsp vanilla extract

Method

1. Whizz the fruit, seeds and vanilla extract briefly in a small food processor until smooth. Tip into a bowl and chill until ready to serve. The jam will keep in the fridge for up to 5 days.

Tiramisu

·······················

Makes 8 portions

Per serving: Total carbs 12 g, fibre 2.6 g, protein 8.5 g, fat 27 g, 333 kcal

hen Giancarlo Caldesi was
agnosed with type 2 diabetes,
e and his wife Katie knew that
ey would have to develop a new
w-carb version of their most
pular of desserts – tiramisu.
glorious Italian classic, it took
onths of experimentation by
e Caldesi cookery school expert
stry chef, Sefano Borella, to
rfect this version which has
ly 12 g of carbs per portion!

gredients

r the sponge

3 large Medjool dates, pitted and
finely chopped

2 tbsp very hot water

3 medium free-range eggs, whites
and yolks separated

1 tsp vanilla extract

75 g (2¾ oz) ground almonds

1 tsp baking powder

the cream

1 large Medjool date, pitted and
finely chopped

2 tbsp very hot water

200 g (7 oz) mascarpone

2 medium free-range eggs, whites
and yolks separated

1 tsp vanilla extract

- 150 ml (¼ pint) whipping cream

To serve

- 100 ml (3½ fl oz) cold strong coffee
- 3 tbsp Marsala or brandy
- 2 tbsp cocoa powder, to dust

Method

1. Preheat the oven to 190°C (375°F, gas mark 5) and line a 20-cm (8-inch) round cake tin with parchment paper.

2. To make the sponge, soften the dates in the hot water in a mug while mashing them with a fork. Use a spoon to push the softened dates through a sieve into a bowl, discarding the skins.

3. Add the egg yolks and vanilla extract to the date mixture and whisk together. Sift in the ground almonds and baking powder and stir everything together so it is well combined.

4. In another bowl, whisk the egg whites with clean, dry beaters until they hold their shape as stiff peaks. Now gently fold the egg whites into the egg yolk mixture with a large spoon until it is all just one colour.

5. Pour this mixture into the cake tin and bake in the oven for 18–20 minutes or until it is firm to the touch and lightly browned. Remove the cake from the oven and allow to cool on a wire rack.

6. Once cooled, cut the cake into finger-sized pieces and set aside.

7. To make the cream, soften the date in the hot water as above. Sieve as before, discarding the skin, into a bowl and add the mascarpone, egg yolks and vanilla extract. Now using either an electric mixer or a handheld whisk, whisk the mixture until it is well combined and creamy.

8. Whip the whipping cream until it forms soft peaks and gently fold into the mascarpone mixture with a spoon or a spatula.

9. Whisk the egg whites with clean, dry beaters until they form soft peaks and lightly fold into the cream mixture.

10. To serve, mix the coffee and marsala together in a small bowl. Dip the sponge fingers briefly into the liquid and divide them between 8 small serving glasses. Divide the cream between the 8 glasses and chill in the fridge for at least an hour and up to 24 hours. Serve dusted with cocoa powder.

This recipe is taken from: *The Reverse Your Diabetes Cookbook: Lose Weight and Eat to Beat Type 2 Diabetes* by Katie and Giancarlo Caldesi published by Kyle Books (2020).

Mrs P's Low-Carb Trifle

....

Serves 8 or more portions

Per serving: Total carbs 15.8 g, fibre 2 g, protein 8 g, fat 22 g, 287 kcal
The carb content for the sponge alone is 2.5 g carbs per slice,
based on 14 slices, using 20 g muscovado sugar

Emma Porter and I published *The Low-Carb Diabetes Cookbook* in 2018 and Emma's recipes were and still re widely admired. This is her low-carb version of that family favourite.

Emma says,'The quantities will make 20-slice sponge which can then be ut into fingers. Personally, I would dd only half of the sponge to the ecipe, but if you like it particularly akey then by all means add the lot.'

Ingredients

For the sponge

- 150 g (5¼ oz) ground almonds (if you are nut-intolerant use ground golden flaxseed)
- 200 ml (6¾ fl oz) full-fat milk
- 2 large free-range eggs, beaten
- 1 tsp baking powder
- 20 g (¾ oz) muscovado sugar or sweetener alternative (1 tbsp sweetener max)

For the fruit

- 400 g (14 oz) thawed frozen fruit plus 50 ml (1¾ fl oz) of the juice from the thawed fruit
- 3 tbsp chia seeds

Or

- 400 g (14 oz) thawed frozen fruit plus 150 ml (5 fl oz) jelly (I use a sugar-free strawberry packet. Follow the instructions then use just 150 ml (5 fl oz) for this dessert. Chill the rest to have another time)

For the custard

- 150 ml (5 fl oz) double cream
- 2 large free-range egg yolks (use the best eggs you can – the more orange the yolk, the better the custard)
- 50 ml (1¾ fl oz) full-fat milk
- 1 tsp vanilla extract
- 1–1½ tsp sweetener (I recommend a powdered sweetener)

For the cream

- 250 ml (8½ fl oz) double or whipping cream

To serve

- 20 g (¾ oz) 85% cocoa chocolate, grated
- 50 g (1¾ oz) raspberries or blueberries

Method

For the sponge

1. Preheat the oven to 180°C (350°F, gas mark 4) and line a 20-cm (8-inch) round cake tin with parchment paper.

2. Combine the ground almonds, milk, eggs and baking powder in a bowl. Add the sugar or sweetener to the mix last. If you are happy to, taste the raw batter to test the sweetness, adjusting carefully.

3. Bake for 25 minutes until a knife put through the middle of the sponge comes out clean.

4. Remove from the tin and allow to cool on a wire rack before cutting into slices and then into fingers.

5. In a large glass bowl combine the thawed fruit, the cake (I use 220 g / 7¾ oz of the baked cake, so about half) and chia seeds. Pour over the juice. Alternatively, instead of the juice and chia, you can add the jelly.

6. Pop into the fridge to set for 1 hour, but it will need 6–8 hours or so if you have used the jelly.

For the custard

1. Whisk the cream until it thickens. Whisk the egg yolks in a separate bowl until they are thick and pale.

2. Put the milk and vanilla extract into a heavy-bottomed saucepan and warm over a low heat. Add the whisked cream and, little by little, the sweetener. Have a taste until you are happy with the sweetness.

3. Continue to warm slowly while stirring continuously with a wooden spoon until the custard is thick enough to coat the back of the spoon. This will take around 8 minutes. Test it by running a finger through the custard on the spoon: if it leaves a straight, clear line, it's ready. Boiling point is the enemy once you have added the eggs, so always keep the temperature of the custard just below the boil. If it boils, the eggs will begin to separate.

4. Allow to cool before pouring on top of the set fruit element of the trifle.

For the cream

1. Whip the cream with a hand whisk until it thickens and carefully spoon on top of the custard. I find putting 5 or 6 dollops down and then using the back of a fork the easiest way to spread it.

2. Pop back in the fridge for an hour or so before serving. Sprinkle over the grated chocolate and raspberries or blueberries.

This recipe is taken from Emma's book in progress, which is destined for her website and is taught in her cookery classes to much acclaim. You can see more of Emma's recipes at TheLowCarbKitchen.co.uk

Useful websites and further reading

Websites

www.amclowcarb.com – The website of a GP surgery in London that has done all the hard work for you and collected a variety of useful resources in one place.

www.carbsandcals.com – The home of the famous Carbs & Cals books and app.

www.diabetes.co.uk – A UK website run by a commercial company, not to be confused with the charity Diabetes UK (see next entry). They have long supported a low-carb approach and pioneered the Low Carb Program (www.lowcarbprogram.com). It is home to many very useful forums where you can get sensible advice and information from other people with diabetes.

www.diabetes.org.uk – The website of the national diabetes charity known as Diabetes UK. It contains a wealth of information, although I find that much of the dietary information is confusing. They sometimes seem ambivalent about low-carb approaches, and suggest it is an option that is no better or worse than other approaches.

www.dietdoctor.com – A Swedish website (in English) that has huge amounts of resources, information and recipes about using a low-carb lifestyle to improve your health.

www.drdavidcavan.com – My website that lets you know what I have been getting up to, gives details of my books and how to arrange a consultation. You can also get in touch with me to tell me how you get on after reading the book.

www.fatismyfriend.co.uk – A blog set up by Dr Joanne McCormack who is a GP in Warrington in the north-west of England. It includes loads of useful information and some recipes. She runs free courses to help people lose weight and reverse their diabetes with a low-carb diet.

www.lowcarbkitchen.co.uk – Here, you will find a wealth of invaluable information and great recipes created by Emma Porter, who wrote the recipes in the *Low Carb Diabetes Cookbook*. She has type 1 diabetes and understands how food affects blood glucose levels.

www.HealthResults.com – Health Results is a UK preventative healthcare organization. Their website includes free articles, videos, resources and recipes for reversing type 2 diabetes.

www.newforestpcn.co.uk – Another great collection of resources from GPs in my neck of the woods in the New Forest in southern England.

www.phcuk.org – The website of the Public Health Collaboration, with information about low-carb research, resources including Dr Unwin's 'sugar infographics' and details of the ambassador programme.

Books

The 30 Minute Diabetes Cookbook: Eat to Beat Diabetes with 100 Easy Low-Carb Recipes by Katie and Giancarlo Caldesi

The 4 Pillar Plan by Dr Rangan Chatterjee – A helpful lifestyle guide that includes excellent advice about how to eat well, reduce stress and improve sleep.

The 8-Week Blood Sugar Diet by Dr Michael Mosley – A guide to using real food to achieve rapid weight loss on a low-calorie diet.

Carbs & Cals Carb & Calorie Counter by Chris Cheyette and Yello Balolia – The bible of carb counting.

Carbs & Cals Very Low Calorie Recipes & Meal Plans by Chris Cheyette and Yello Balolia – For people who wish to follow an 800-calorie diet.

Carbs & Cals World Foods by Salma Mehar, Dr Joan St John, Chris Cheyette and Yello Balolia – Provides information on carbohydrate content of common African, Arabic, Caribbean and South Asian foods.

The Complete Guide to Fasting by Dr Jason Fung and Jimmy Moore – Great practical guide to intermittent fasting.

The Diabetes Weight-Loss Cookbook by Katie and Giancarlo Caldesi – Low-carb recipes to help reverse type 2 diabetes.

The Low-Carb Diabetes Cookbook by Dr David Cavan and Emma Porter – Fantastic recipes created by a person with diabetes.

The Reverse Your Diabetes Cookbook: Lose Weight and Eat to Beat Type 2 Diabetes by Katie and Giancarlo Caldesi

APPENDIX B

BMI chart

To find your BMI, locate where your height and weight intersect; your BMI is listed is in the square.

WEIGHT

	lbs	90	100	110	120	130	140	150	160	170	180	190	200	210	220	230	240	250	260	270	280	290
	kgs	41	45	50	54	59	64	68	73	77	82	86	91	95	100	104	109	113	118	122	127	132
ft/in	cm																					
4'8"	142.2	20	22	25	27	29	31	34	36	38	40	43	45	47	49	52	54	56	58	61	63	65
4'9"	144.7	19	22	24	26	28	30	32	35	37	39	41	43	45	48	50	52	54	56	58	61	63
4'10"	147.3	19	21	23	25	27	29	31	33	36	38	40	42	44	46	48	50	52	54	56	59	61
4'11"	149.8	18	20	22	24	26	28	30	32	34	36	38	40	42	44	46	48	51	53	55	57	59
5'0"	152.4	18	20	21	23	25	27	29	31	33	35	37	39	41	43	45	47	49	51	53	55	57
5'1"	154.9	17	19	21	23	25	26	28	30	32	34	36	38	40	42	43	45	47	49	51	53	55
5'2"	157.4	16	18	20	22	24	26	27	29	31	33	35	37	38	40	42	44	46	48	49	51	53
5'3"	160.0	16	18	19	21	23	25	27	28	30	32	34	35	37	39	41	43	44	46	48	50	51
5'4"	162.5	15	17	19	21	22	24	26	27	29	31	33	34	36	38	39	41	43	45	46	48	50
5'5"	165.1	15	17	18	20	22	23	25	27	28	30	32	33	35	37	38	40	42	43	45	47	48
5'6"	167.6	15	16	18	19	21	23	24	26	27	29	31	32	34	36	37	39	40	42	44	45	47
5'7"	170.1	14	16	17	19	20	22	24	25	27	28	30	31	33	34	36	38	39	41	42	44	45
5'8"	172.7	14	15	17	18	20	21	23	24	26	27	29	30	32	33	35	37	38	40	41	43	44
5'9"	175.2	13	15	16	18	19	21	22	24	25	27	28	30	31	33	34	35	37	38	40	41	43
5'10"	177.8	13	14	16	17	19	20	22	23	24	26	27	29	30	32	33	34	36	37	39	40	42
5'11"	180.3	13	14	15	17	18	20	21	22	24	25	27	28	29	31	32	33	35	36	38	39	40
6'0"	182.8	12	14	15	16	18	19	20	22	23	24	26	27	28	30	31	33	34	35	37	38	39
6'1"	185.4	12	13	15	16	17	18	20	21	22	24	25	26	28	29	30	32	33	34	36	37	38
6'2"	187.9	12	13	14	15	17	18	19	21	22	23	24	26	27	28	30	31	32	33	35	36	37
6'3"	190.5	11	13	14	15	16	18	19	20	21	23	24	25	26	28	29	30	31	33	34	35	36
6'4"	193.0	11	12	13	15	16	17	18	19	21	22	23	24	26	27	28	29	30	32	33	34	35
6'5"	195.5	11	12	13	14	15	17	18	19	20	21	23	24	25	26	27	28	30	31	32	33	34
6'6"	198.1	10	12	13	14	15	16	17	18	20	21	22	23	24	25	27	28	29	30	31	32	34
6'7"	200.6	10	11	12	14	15	16	17	18	19	20	21	23	24	25	26	27	28	29	30	32	33
6'8"	203.2	10	11	12	13	14	15	16	18	19	20	21	22	23	24	25	26	27	29	30	31	32
6'9"	205.7	10	11	12	13	14	15	16	17	18	19	20	21	24	24	25	26	27	28	29	30	31
6'10"	208.2	9	10	12	13	14	15	16	17	18	19	20	21	22	23	24	25	26	27	28	29	30
6'11"	210.8	9	10	11	12	13	14	15	16	17	18	19	20	21	22	23	25	26	27	28	29	30

HEIGHT

Underweight · Healthy · Overweight · Obese · Extremely Obese

← REDUCED RISK INCREASED RISK →

Source: bmicalculatoruk.com (accessed 1 September 2021).

Endnotes

1 https://www.diabetes.org.uk/type-2-diabetes (accessed 17 August 2021).

2 M.C. Riddle et al. 'Consensus report: definition and interpretation of remission in type 2 diabetes', *Diabetologia*, 2021, https://doi.org/10.1007/s00125-021-05542-z.

3 D.M. Nathan, 'International Expert Committee report on the role of the A1C assay in the diagnosis of diabetes', *Diabetes Care*, vol. 32, no. 7, 2009, pp. 1327–1334.

4 T. Watson, 'Tom Watson MP in UK Parliament – on the importance of #LCHF diet for health and reversing Diabetes!' [video], YouTube, 2 March 2019, https://www.youtube.com/watch?v=rGMrgXbNSCA (accessed 17 August 2021).

5 T. Watson, *Downsizing*, Kyle Books, 2020, p. 121.

6 S. Lim, J. Hyun Bae, H.-S. Kwon and M.A. Nauck, 'COVID-19 and diabetes mellitus: from pathophysiology to clinical management', *Nature Reviews Endocrinology*, vol. 17, 2021, pp. 11–30, https://doi.org/10.1038/s41574-020-00435-4.

7 https://www.nhs.uk/conditions/diabetic-eye-screening (accessed 17 August 2021).

8 International Diabetes Federation, *IDF Diabetes Atlas*, 9th edition, 2019, https://www.diabetesatlas.org/en/ (accessed 17 August 2021).

9 S.H. Ley, O. Hamdy, V. Mohan and F.B. Hu, 'Prevention and management of type 2 diabetes: dietary components and nutritional strategies', *The Lancet*, vol. 383, 2014, pp. 1999–2007.

10 D. Pell et al., 'Changes in soft drinks purchased by British households associated with the UK soft drinks industry levy: controlled interrupted time series analysis', *British Medical Journal*, vol. 372, no. 254, 2021.

11 UK Prospective Diabetes Study, https://www.dtu.ox.ac.uk/ukpds/ (accessed 18 August 2021).

12 Diabetes Prevention Program Research Group, 'Reduction in the incidence of type 2 diabetes with lifestyle intervention or metformin', *New England Journal of Medicine*, vol. 346, 2002, pp. 393–403.

13 J. Lindstrom et al., 'The Finnish Diabetes Prevention Study (DPS): lifestyle intervention and 3-year results on diet and physical activity', *Diabetes Care*, vol. 26, no. 12, 2003, pp. 3230–3236.

14 E.L. Lim et al., 'Reversal of type 2 diabetes: normalisation of beta cell function in association with decreased pancreas and liver triacylglycerol', *Diabetologia*, vol. 54, no. 10, 2011, pp. 2506–2514.

15 S. Hallberg, 'Dr Sarah Hallberg – Type 2 Diabetes Reversal' [video], YouTube, 31 October 2018, https://www.

youtube.com/watch?v=JUuHrBwsJ2s (accessed 18 August 2021).

16 M. Lean et al., 'Durability of a primary care-led weight-management intervention for remission of type 2 diabetes: 2-year results of the DiRECT open-label, cluster-randomised trial', *Lancet Diabetes and Endocrinology*, vol. 7, no. 5, 2019, pp. 344–355.

17 S.J. Hallberg et al., 'Effectiveness and safety of a novel care model for the management of type 2 diabetes at 1 year: an open-label, non-randomized, controlled study', *Diabetes Therapy*, vol. 9, no. 2, 2018, pp. 583–612.

18 D. Unwin et al., 'Insights from a general practice service evaluation supporting a lower carbohydrate diet in patients with type 2 diabetes mellitus and prediabetes: a secondary analysis of routine clinic data including HbA1c, weight and prescribing over 6 years', *BMJ Nutrition, Prevention & Health*, 2020, e000072, doi:10.1136/bmjnph-2020-000072.

19 T.D.R. Hockaday, J.M. Hockaday, J.I. Mann and R.C. Turner, 'Prospective comparison of modified fat high carbohydrate with standard low carbohydrate dietary advice in the treatment of diabetes: one year follow up study', *British Journal of Nutrition*, vol. 39, no. 2, 1978, pp. 357–362.

20 R.W. Simpson et al., 'Improved glucose control in maturity-onset diabetes treated with a high carbohydrate modified fat diet', *British Medical Journal*, vol. 1, no. 6180, 1979, pp. 1753–1756.

21 SACN, 'Lower carbohydrate diets for adults with type 2 diabetes', Scientific Advisory Committee on Nutrition, May 2021, https://www.gov.uk/government/publications/sacn-report-lower-carbohydrate-diets-for-type-2-diabetes (accessed 18 August 2021).

22 M. Dehghan et al., 'Association of fats and carbohydrate intake with cardiovascular disease and mortality in 18 countries from five continents (PURE): a prospective cohort study', *The Lancet*, vol. 390, issue 10107, 2017, pp. 2050–2062.

23 R. Estruch et al., 'Primary prevention of cardiovascular disease with a Mediterranean diet', *New England Journal of Medicine*, vol. 368, 2013, pp. 1279–1290.

24 M.S. Farvid et al., 'Dairy food intake and all-cause cardiovascular disease and cancer mortality: The Golestan cohort study', *American Journal of Epidemiology*, vol. 185, no. 8, 2017, pp. 697–711.

25 https://www.freestylelibre.co.uk/libre/ (accessed 18 August 2021).

26 W.H. Polonsky et al., 'Structured self-monitoring of blood glucose significantly reduces A1C levels in poorly controlled, noninsulin-treated type 2 patients: results from the Structured Testing Program study', *Diabetes Care*, vol. 34, no. 2, 2011, pp. 262–267.

27 S.D. Phinney and J.S. Volek, *The Art and Science of Low Carbohydrate Living*, Beyond Obesity LLC, 2011.

28 NHS, 'Exercise', 2019, https://www.nhs.uk/live-well/exercise/ (accessed 18 August 2021).

29 J.N. Morris et al., 'Coronary heart-disease and physical activity of work', *The Lancet*, vol. 262, no. 6795, 1953, pp. 1053–1057.

30 H. Rasmus et al., 'Metabolic responses to reduced daily steps in healthy nonexercising men', *JAMA*, vol. 299, no. 11, 2008, pp. 1261–1263.

31 A.A. Laverty, J.S. Mindell, E.A. Webb and C. Millett, 'Active travel to work and cardiovascular risk factors in the United Kingdom', *American Journal of Preventive Medicine*, vol. 45, no. 3, 2013, pp. 282–288.

32 N. Genevieve et al., 'Breaks in sedentary time: beneficial associations

with metabolic risk', *Diabetes Care*, vol. 31, no. 4, 2008, pp. 661–666.

33 A. Grøntved and F.B. Hu, 'Television viewing and risk of type 2 diabetes, cardiovascular disease, and all-cause mortality: a meta-analysis', *JAMA*, vol. 305, no. 23, 2011, pp. 2448–2455.

34 A.R. Cooper et al., 'Sedentary time breaks in sedentary time and metabolic variables in people with newly diagnosed type 2 diabetes', *Diabetologia*, vol. 55, no. 3, 2021, pp. 589–599.

35 https://www.parkrun.org.uk/ (accessed 18 August 2021).

36 R. De Cabo and M.P. Mattson, 'Effects of intermittent fasting on health, aging and disease', *New England Journal of Medicine*, vol. 381, 2019, pp. 2541–2551.

37 https://www.carbsandcals.com (accessed 19 August 2021). Carbs & Cals are a very useful series of books to help with different aspects of carbohydrate and calorie counting. They include: *Carb & Calorie Counter, Very Low Calorie Recipes & Meal Plans* and the *World Foods* book that includes Asian, African and Caribbean foods. The app is also very useful.

38 https://foodaddictioninstitute.org/ for-food-addicts/ (accessed 19 August 2021); https://www.bittensaddiction. com/en/patients/help-available/ (accessed 19 August 2021).

39 C. Murdoch et al., 'Adapting diabetes medication for low carbohydrate management of type 2 diabetes', *British Journal of General Practice*, vol. 69, no. 684, 2019, pp. 360–361.

40 V. Singh and B. Garg, 'Insulin resistance and depression: relationship and treatment implications', *Journal of Mental Health and Human Behaviour*, vol. 24, no. 1, 2019, pp. 4–7.

41 L. Lachance and D. Ramsey, 'Food, mood and brain health: implications for the modern clinician', *Missouri Medicine*, vol. 112, no. 2, 2015, pp. 111–115.

42 M.P. White et al., 'Spending at least 120 minutes a week in nature is associated with good health and wellbeing', *Scientific Reports*, vol. 9, article 7730, 2019.

43 A. Mullens, 'Is low carb and keto safe during pregnancy?', Diet Doctor, 17 June 2021, https://www.dietdoctor. com/low-carb/pregnancy (accessed 20 August 2021).

44 QRISK3 calculator for risk of heart attack or stroke: https://www.qrisk.org/ three/ (accessed 20 August 2021).

45 L. Saslow, C. Summers, J.E. Aikens, D.J. Unwin, 'Outcomes of a digitally delivered low carbohydrate type 2 diabetes self-management program: 1 year results of a single-arm longitudinal study', *JMIR Diabetes*, vol. 3, no. 3, 2018, e12.

46 E.L. Lim et al., 'Reversal of type 2 diabetes: normalisation of beta cell function in association with decreased pancreas and liver triacylglycerol', *Diabetologia*, vol. 54, no. 10, 2011, pp. 2506–2514.

Acknowledgements

There are many individuals who have been instrumental in shaping my journey since the publication of *Reverse Your Diabetes*, and who have thereby helped shape this book.

They include all those who took the trouble to contact me after reading *Reverse Your Diabetes*, to tell me that they managed to do just that. Special thanks are due to everyone who allowed me to include their story in this book. I have no doubt that their words will be hugely encouraging to others as they embark on their own journey to reverse their condition. One of them is Dan Parker, a former advertising executive who marketed junk food; he has been instrumental in helping me understand the tactics used by the food industry and his erstwhile colleagues to encourage us to eat unhealthy food. Another is Eddy Marshall, who, after reversing his own diabetes, set up a programme in 2017 to help others in his area do the same. He provided me with early feedback on his programme, just as I was setting up a Diabetes Reversal Programme in Bermuda, at the invitation of Dr Stanley James. He and his team at the Premier Health and Wellness Center, Sara Bosch de Noya and Debbie Jones of the Bermuda Diabetes Association, and Joan Everett, a former colleague from the Bournemouth Diabetes and Endocrine Centre, were all instrumental in its success. As was Dr

Daniel Katambo who then took it to his native Kenya and is now working with colleagues elsewhere in Africa to promote reversal of type 2 diabetes in their countries.

Thanks also to the many colleagues who shared their ideas and experiences of diabetes reversal and helped shape my own thinking. Notable among them are Dr Sarah Hallberg of Virta Health in the US and Dr David Unwin from the UK. Along the way I have learnt so much more about nutrition (barely covered in medical training) and many other aspects of human health and psychology. I have also learnt about the impact of food addiction, and am very grateful to Heidi Giaever, who is an expert in the field and contributed significantly to the section on food addiction in Chapter 12.

This book would not have been possible without the hard grind behind the scenes of my literary agent, Jonathan Hayden, and the team at Atlantic Books who have been very supportive and patient with me throughout the writing process. I am doubly grateful to Jonathan as he has produced some mouth-watering low-carb recipes for the final section. Special thanks to Katie and Giancarlo Caldesi and to Emma Porter, all established low-carb recipe writers, who kindly and generously contributed their own recipes. As always, my wife Mary has been constantly supportive, sharing the journey (often literally) and offering many excellent ideas that fed their way into the book.

Index

Index

Index

Index